My OWN Weigh

Steve Taylor

My OWN Weigh

By Steve Taylor

Acknowledgements

It takes a lot more than just putting ideas down on paper to write a book. If it were that easy, more people would do it. It also takes a lot more work than any author ever anticipates. That's why most authors seek help to get a book published. As much as I would like to think otherwise, I am no different.

I was fortunate to have two trusted friends and colleagues help me bring to life my battles, anguish, and victories in these pages… and for that I am very grateful. They helped make this project even more fun and a work of pride. I want to extend my appreciation to them both.

First my thanks goes to Cyndee Davis who encouraged me to rewrite the original book and gave me ideas to help expand it into a more useful tool for my readers. She also designed and developed my website, creating a warm and welcoming place for you to come and be a part of a community with others who have experienced similar weight loss journeys. Cyndee is a marketing consultant who can be contacted at www.ocavancopy.com.

Next, my extreme gratitude goes to Christine Butler, whose painstaking patience and perseverance have helped me produce this book through restructuring, editing, formatting, and publishing to get this tool into your hands. Her support, commitment, endurance, and professionalism will never be forgotten. She can be reached for her marketing expertise via her website, www.TheButlerWroteIt.com.

Introduction

In writing My OWN Weigh, I have squeezed fifty years of emotional and physical suffering into this short book. My primary purpose for writing about my journey and what I discovered is to provide hope and inspiration for my fellow overeaters and emotional eaters. I do, however, want you to share my beliefs of what I discovered, the myth from the truth about the diet industry. There are, after all, billions of dollars being scrambled for by enterprising, ambitious, well meaning, knowledgeable, and sometimes unfortunately, less than honest opportunists.

All the diets work. No one diet is right for everybody. Emotional Eating is the main culprit for a lot of people really struggling with weight loss. These are some of the issues I address in these following chapters. I hope it is an easy enjoyable read for you and that you feel like you got your money's worth.

In order to make it as enjoyable and informative for you as possible, I have some suggestions on how you may want to approach the material within. The book features three different sections.

First is my story, a compelling tale of a fifty plus year struggle with morbid obesity. I also walk you through the pain and frustration of losing 1000 pounds over the years.

The second section of the book is the heart of the book in the sense that it tells how I did it by detailing what type of eating plan and exercise finally produced long-term results. It presents the physical part of how I overcame a lifelong search for the "right diet", by creating "The Three Bears Diet." I also give my opinion of some of the many, many other diets I tried, what I think about supplements, and answer some of the most frequently asked questions of me about this widely confusing, contradictory and contested industry, the diet industry.

You will receive some food education 101. I also touch briefly on exercising, but since I am not a trainer, it's important for you to find out what exercise routine works for you.

If Section Two is the heart of the book, then Section Three is the soul of the book. While Section Two addresses the physical part (diet and exercise) of weight loss, Section Three talks about what almost no other diet books address, the psychological part of overeating, EMOTIONAL EATING. While others simply say you have to change your habits and develop a new lifestyle, this section describes your problem, the diagnosis, and gives you a blue print on how to solve it. Therefore, the prognosis is, "You can be cured!"

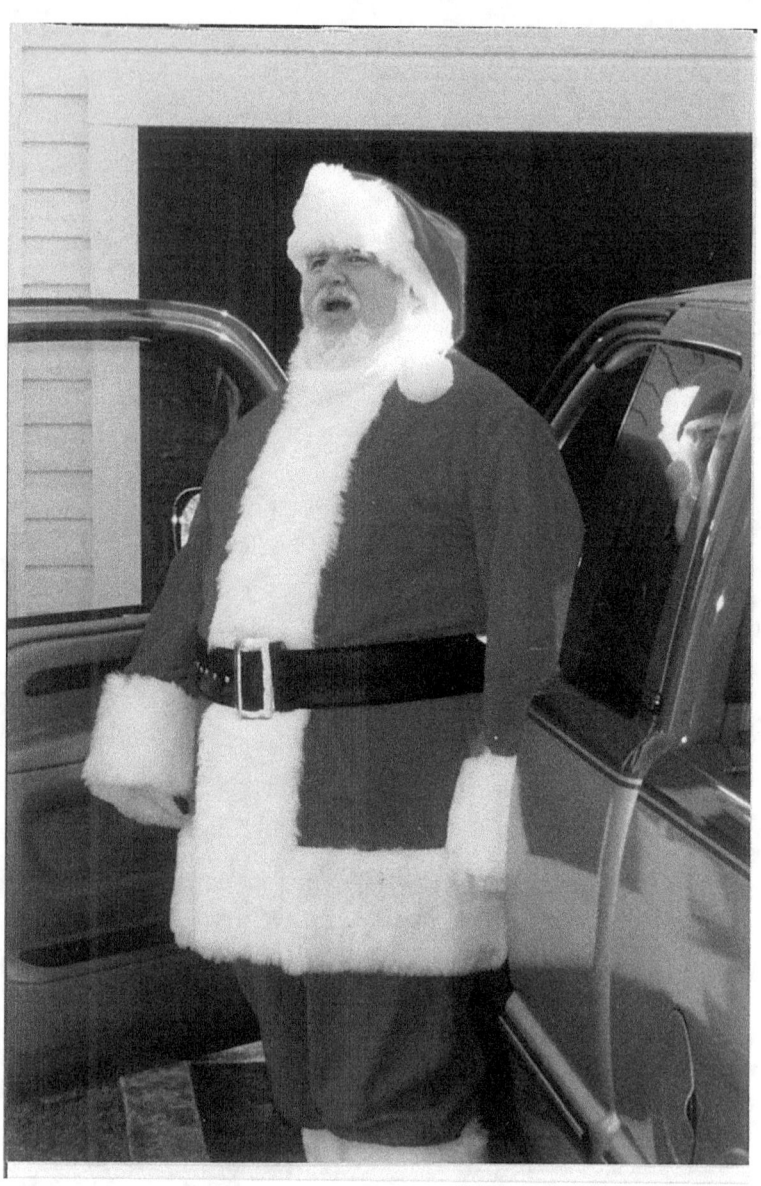

Ode To A Fat Boy by Steve Taylor

Ode to a fat boy playing Santa Claus.

Is he really a jolly fat man

Or just supporting a cause

Is he laughing on the outside

And crying on the in

And wishing with a fervor

That he was really thin

Oh the many diets of which he did partake

But somehow falling short of the final goal to make.

Oh diet oh new diet can't you make me thin

When I am fat life is so grim

How can I expel this obsession this compulsive overeating

Arrest my mind, body, and soul, of this constant beating

One day an epiphany arose a special treasured gem

The feeling was so powerful

He knew it's not a whim

Maybe it was not what he was eating

But what was eating him.

Section 1 – My Story

Chapter One
The Purpose and Meaningfulness of My OWN Weigh

They say in everyone there is a book. This book, *My OWN Weigh*, was never on my mind until I accomplished a lifetime goal of losing a lot of weight and keeping it off. The purpose of this book is to let you know that if you suffer, there is hope for you. That is worth repeating. If you suffer from obesity or morbid obesity, there is hope for you. I demonstrate this to you by sharing my trials and tribulations and how overcoming them gave me a new purpose and meaningfulness in life.

In viewing my journey you will discover some secrets that will help you lose weight. These secrets will in all probability change your life. That is why I am being so open about my life because I think I have a chance to help you get on track to change yours.

Don't you believe for a second that people cannot change. Certain personality traits will not change but when you change your attitude, oh what a difference you will feel in yourself that will transform your thinking and others' thinking towards you.

Although you will learn some secrets from this book, there is one secret that everyone has to discover for him or herself. I can help you search for it but you will have to be the one that finds it. What is it? It's deciding that you have hit bottom, that it's time to stop digging and be willing to change. Inside you and all of us there is an answer. We all just have to decide when the pain becomes too great and therefore muster the courage to change.

If you have already made that decision to be willing to change, you will be successful. So let's just suppose for a minute that you have hit bottom and are willing to look at a different way of approaching weight loss. You probably made that decision because like me you have been on all or most of the diets, and like me maybe you lost 100 pounds or more on some of them. But did you keep it off? That's all right. I already know the answer. You put it back on and maybe added a few extra pounds. Take a peek into my life. See if you can identify.

Chapter Two
Steve's Story

My first realization for me that I was fat or different was in Elementary School. My memory serves me as being in either the second or third grade. That would translate to an age of about seven or eight years. We were having what was then called recess, a supposedly fun time. We were being taught square dancing. When it became time to hook up with this pretty little girl in my class she reacted unfavorably. I was rejected. She wanted no part of this fat boy. I remember the hurt, a feeling of being less than my peers. Little did I know then that feeling less than others would repeatedly occur over much of my life.

Through the rest of elementary school I was conscious of my weight. I cannot imagine this being done today but in the 50's they weighed us at school. I don't remember the teachers shouting out the weights of every student to the rest of the class; however, I don't recall much privacy either. I think it was in the third grade that I weighed 110 pounds. Word got around.

At the end of elementary school or what is now the start of middle school, my parents took me to the doctor. I remember having a metabolism test that showed yes, my metabolism was a little slow but it was really not abnormal. The doctor put me on a diet. I really don't remember much about it except there were instructions not to eat sweets and not to eat between meals. We shot for a target of five pounds per month. When weigh-in time came I knew what the results would be. I had been cheating. I could not do without the candy. My parents were disappointed. I felt worthless. I think it made a mark on me. It made me feel once again less than and unconfident.

When I reached Middle School two of my buddies and I were paraded on stage in front of the general assembly; i.e., the whole school. Our football coach said, "Look at these boys, I am going to have them in shape." This now would be unfathomable. Can you imagine the lawsuits? Actually, then it wasn't so bad. Although it embarrassed the hell out of us we laugh about it to this day. One of those guys retired as head of a very successful engineering firm, and the other as a circuit judge. Although it had no lasting mark, it is just not something a seventh grader should have to endure. Being a fat kid affects all of your life including your home life.

As an early teenager, I remember my mother used to cook a roast in a crockpot. One day I decided to sample tonight's dinner. I had a sample, and then another sample, and then another sample, and the sampling continued until the roast was almost gone. Can you imagine my mother's dismay when she arrived to prepare the evening meal? At first she was angry but later laughed and joked with her friends that I had eaten a whole roast. Come on, Mom! There was a little bit left. It hurt me that Mother told her friends. I felt guilty and gluttonous. That roast, that tender succulent derivative of heaven, producing those orgasmic like sensations of the eating process, I just could not stop eating it.

My weight was an albatross I carried with me the rest of my school years until my senior year in high school. I had become very interested in the opposite sex, something by the way that has stayed with me. Unfortunately, fat boys finished last in the girlfriend race. I put my blinders on and became focused and determined, one meal a day, lunch at school and that was it.

A good friend who was a great football player, who later played at Georgia Tech, was cheering me on. We would go downtown and weigh on those big scales in front of that furniture store. I lost 70 to 80 pounds and got my weight down to around 225 pounds. Little did I know then that would be only the first time of many times that I would have a major weight loss only to regain it. In fact, this may sound incredible, but I believe it to be an accurate estimate that over my lifetime I have lost almost 1,000 pounds. There have been at least five occasions when I have lost a lot of weight only to regain it. Then there have been at least a dozen or so spurts of dieting where I have lost 20 or more pounds. In the next chapter, I take you through my weight loss journey. My intent is not to bore you with a story of every diet run I made. I do want to impress upon you how serious and deep-rooted my problem was and how I overcame it. This hopefully will show you that if I overcame it so can you.

Always a big fan of Johnny Carson and *The Tonight Show*, I was watching Buddy Hackett, a very funny man talking about a very serious subject, weight control. I suppose this was sometime in the 60s. Like so many of us, Buddy had the yo-yo syndrome. He would lose weight then gain it back, up and down and up and down. In his conversation with Johnny, Buddy mentioned something I will never forget. He said there was a little button that automatically triggered to ignite his hunger. He did not know why or when it was going to happen. This is a paraphrasing of Buddy's comments but the message hit home. I had experienced that many times, remember the pot roast cooked in the crockpot? I did not know how, why, or when my insatiable appetite would kick into overdrive.

Eating disorders are progressive meaning it gets worse if not curtailed or arrested. I kept picking up unnecessary baggage. That 225 pounds I weighed when I started to college in 1961 had almost doubled by 1998. That was the year my all time high was recorded at a Weight Watchers facility of 440 pounds. Keep in mind that over this long stretch of time I had lost a lot of weight only to gain it back and then some. That is a disease! That is an eating disorder!

Through most of my business career I was in sales. I was a good salesman. I have also been told that I am intelligent and creative. Therefore, I do possess some God given talents. Probably the best gift I was given was the ability to act. This acting showed a side of me but not the total person. I was miserable with the way

I looked and felt. This misery translated to other people like my wife. So not only was I miserable but I was making her miserable as well. I am saddened by the fact that Judy, my wife who died of cancer, never got to see me lose this weight.

Although I was a good salesman you can imagine how much my weight hurt my career. From my first job out of college with General Electric to my advertising career, I never saw any 400-pound executives.

I use to hate the Waffle House, but not because of the food and service, they were great. It was those little rigid built in booths. Occasionally someone would suggest a business meeting there and I would dread it. It is embarrassing to have to pull up a chair to one of those booths.

I remember one particular client I had who I visited frequently. He was on the second floor after a steep flight of stairs. The office was located at the top of the stairs and there were a lot of people going in and out. What if just as I got to the top of the stairs breathing heavily the door opened and someone walked out. Normal folks won't relate to this; but I know you that are overweight will. And all of you know there are a lot more personal issues with which we have dealt.

When you are morbidly obese your emotions are constantly at war with your wellness. It has been mentioned a couple of times that my wife died with cancer. There are some of you reading this who have experienced the loss of a spouse. You know how devastating it is. Eight months after her death I had triple by-pass surgery. A couple of years later I made a decision to change. I did everything that I will be recommending in this book; the surrender, the Brain Flush, researched and educated myself on dieting and nutrition, got a plan, and pulled the trigger. Two of my favorite sayings are by Abraham Lincoln and Peter Drucker. To quote Abe Lincoln, "If I had 60 minutes to chop down the tree, I would spend the first twenty minutes sharpening the axe." Peter Drucker said, "The best way to predict the future is to make it happen". Do you have time for one more? "Ready, fire, aim," Fred DeLuca, founder of Subway restaurants.

In other words thoroughly plan, but then apply your knowledge. Get started! You can do it. Go out and bite the stars!

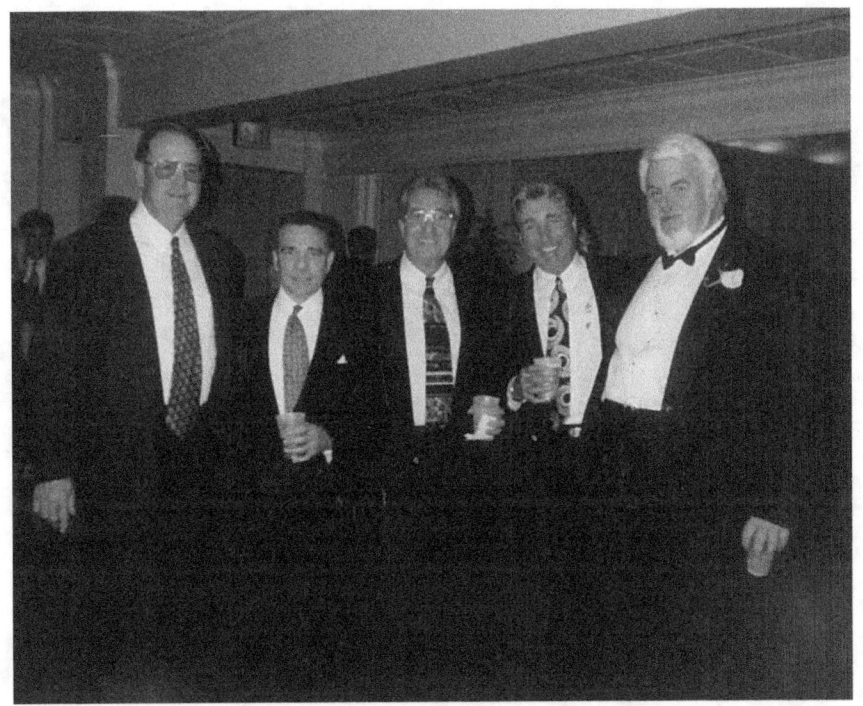

Chapter Three

My Thousand Pound Journey

This is a description of that thousand pounds I lost. I'm writing it out to show you how it actually happened, and to show you that I have always struggled with weight gain the same way you have. And just as you can identify with my ups and downs in weight loss and gain, so you will be able to identify with the SECRET I found that turned it around. So, even though it may seem a bit laborious, please read it all to the very end, because there's something important I want you to see.

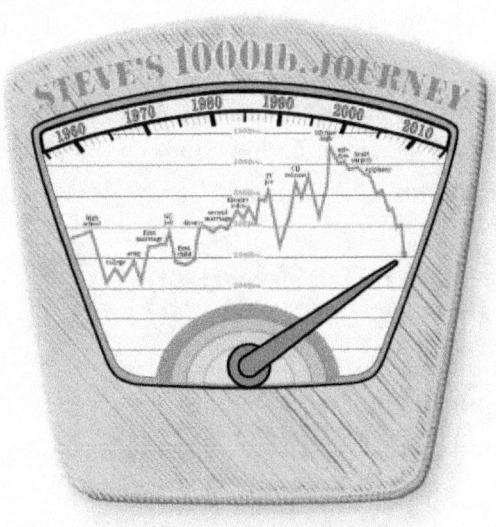

80 pounds in high school

My first major weight loss was in the winter and spring of

1961 when I was a senior in high school. I lost about 80 pounds. I did this with my own self-inflicted diet regime. The only meal I ate every day was my school lunch. My parents marveled at my determination but questioned my methods. They were right to do so. Although I assured them I was fine, I was probably nutritionally deprived. However I did lose weight and graduated from high school weighing 215 to 220 pounds.

Cousin Sonny's diet

After beginning college in the fall of 1961, I gained some weight back. It was then I started Cousin Sonny's diet. We roomed together at Auburn University and ate together at a boarding house. Sonny would not allow me to eat bread, potatoes, and most starches, and of course no sweets. I will never forget after about two weeks and some pleading from me, Sonny let me have a Coca Cola. That was the best Coke I ever had in my life! Remember there were no diet sodas then.

Not only did I give up bread, starches, and sweets, I never ate my usual second servings at the dinner table. On this program I lost about 25 pounds fairly quickly.

Uncle Sam wants YOU to lose weight

Now we are up to a cumulative total of 105 pounds lost. In late 1962 I joined the Army National Guard and went into six-months active service. The first eight weeks were basic training where I lost another 25 pounds. Unfortunately, they were those pounds that I had put back on after dieting in college. This now is early 1963, a total of 130 pounds lost and only 870 more lost pounds to account for in the last fifty years to reach 1000.

After basic training and being assigned to Ft. Gordon, in Augusta, Ga., I proceeded to once again regain some weight, and once again I continued to lose some. I remember going to one meal

12

a day, (sound familiar) a cheeseburger from a burger shop on the base. I stayed out of the chow hall and had about another 25-pound loss. Now I am at 155.

Upon discharge from active duty in July of 1963, I weighed about 215 pounds. But, the yo-yo continued to oscillate. A year and a half later on New Years Eve 1964, I got married. I think I weighed about 265 pounds. Therefore, I had gained 50 pounds in eighteen months. Amazingly, I held that weight until September of 1967. This seemed to break my pattern.

Holding steady

Although I did not lose any weight during this almost three years, I did not gain any either. If I had to guess why, I think I was motivated to look good for interviewing after graduation.

Apparently I looked good enough. I landed a great job with General Electric in the Large Lamp Department, the most profitable division of GE, which all started with Thomas Edison's invention of the light bulb. I really did not appreciate at the time how good a job that was. I began work with them in September of 1967.

Before I take you on another roller coaster ride with me, I think I should explain a few things. First, if you're reading this and you've never had a major problem with food, you probably think this sounds more like fiction. I don't blame you for being a doubting Thomas. You may be wondering, "How can he remember all these gains and losses, and how could he have let this happen?" However, if you've had a major problem with food all of your life, you're probably saying, "This sounds just like me!"

I do have a good memory, but I want you to know that I was, and still am to a certain extent, obsessed with weight. It comes with the territory of an emotional eater who has had a food addiction. I am simply asking for your trust in me. **It's all true.** In fact, the real number is somewhere north of a thousand pounds.

Even I can't remember all of the little 10 or 15 pound losses.

Nearly 300 pounds

Thanks for indulging me. Now back to the journey. In 1968 I had gained enough to have my first flirtation with 300 pounds. The people at GE had not directly accosted me, but I heard things like "you are a big boy." I was very self-conscious of my weight and I knew I had to do something about it. Ah, I heard about a new program that had come on the scene called Weight Watchers. They held meetings where you weighed every week, held you accountable, plus they educated you on food. They also offered an all male meeting, so at least you could just be fat in front of the guys.

Another 60 pounds lost

This all sounded great and I was gung-ho and ready to go. In fact I even joined the YMCA. I was getting up early in the morning before work and going to exercise. Through exercise and this new program called Weight Watchers I lost 60 pounds. Move the total loss to 215 pounds.

My daughter was born March 5, 1969. I weighed about 240 pounds. From March of 1969 until July of 2010, another 41 years, I averaged losing about 20 pounds every year. Here is a quick look at each decade.

From 1974 to 1980, I traveled most of the country. It was difficult not to gain weight, especially when you are not disciplined enough to exercise during your motel stays. At the time I was not.

I went on numerous diets in the 70's including weight watchers several more times, and another one in particular, which was a low fat diet. Back then fat was the real villain. Keep your fat grams to less than 20 or even 10 fat grams per day.

After 1974 I only went south of 300 pounds a couple of times. My average weight in the 70's was somewhere around 310 pounds. I am estimating that I tried 10 or 12 times in the 70's to lose weight. I was always temporarily successful. The key word here being temporarily.

Weight Watchers helps again

I had one major weight loss in the 70's (fifty pounds or more). My best estimate is that I lost about 100 pounds during those other nine years moving the total to 365 pounds. Most of that loss came from visiting my old friends at Weight Watchers, which I joined several times. It always worked, but I always gained the weight back.

A progressive disease

What were the eighties like? As you may imagine, since food addiction is a progressive disease, the eighties were not kind to me. In November of 1979 I began my second marriage. My first one ended in divorce in 1973. I am sure my weight, which caused my unhappiness, indirectly contributed to the collapse of the marriage.

But here I was with my new wife and a second lease on life. When my wife and I began dating, I was only about 270 pounds. That was in 1975. But when we married in November of 1979, the needle had moved above 300. Keep in mind the total is now 365 pounds lost starting with the sixties...but now back to the 80's.

Like a Fiddler on the Roof

Three events stand out in the 80's that were catalysts for some pretty good losses. In 1984, I played Tevye, the lead role in "Fiddler On The Roof" in a theater in Gadsden, Alabama. I lost about 30 pounds before playing that role but still weighed in the low 300s. I also played that same role in a theater in Atlanta, Georgia in May of 1987. I had lost about 20 pounds before that production.

I suppose I weighed around 350 pounds. I was fortunate to receive good reviews for my work. However, one particular reviewer from the Atlanta Constitution said something like this: "As so goes Tevye, so goes Fiddler, and to that end the show is on solid ground." Then I was described as a man of CONSIDERABLE GIRTH and powerful voice. Ouch!! If she noticed how big I was, I bet all of the audience, cast members, directors, etc. noticed too.

There are three tragedies here: First, Tevye is an extremely demanding role. You are on stage in almost every scene. There are a lot of lines to remember; songs demanding a very good vocal range, and a great diversity of emotions are required to be displayed by Tevye. When you get through a performance you feel like you have been to a couple of weddings, a couple of funerals, one exciting football game where your team won, and one disappointing one where your team lost.

You're emotionally drained and not really receptive to subtle ridicule. The second tragedy is that even though I had access to numerous mirrors, even photographs, I did not see myself the same way others did because I did not feel fat inside. That is part of the disease of morbid obesity. The reverse of that would also be true. Anorexic persons do not view themselves as thin.

And lastly, being morbidly obese probably cost me a career in musical theater, the thing I loved most. Of course, it cost me a lot more as well.

Media Sales

In 1987 I left Atlanta to go to work as an account representative for a television station in Alabama. My job was to call on media buyers and direct business and sell them

16

commercials, thereby creating revenue for the station. The media business, as all sales jobs do, puts a premium on looking good off camera as well as on camera. I did not look good. Can you imagine entering a room and being pretty sure you are going to be the biggest one there?

A Liquid Diet

In 1987 the TV station owners traded out (TV advertising for products and services) a weight loss program. This diet involved taking some vitamin supplements and drinking a meal replacement three times a day, no solid food.

I was getting 500 calories per day. The big bonus was getting to dissolve a bouillon cube in hot water and eat it like soup if I wished once per day. My best recollection is that I lost 90 pounds in about five months or less.

This is 140 pounds accounted for in the 80s so far. That weight of course came back and then some. In the other seven years of the 80's, I am saying I probably lost a total of 100 more pounds bringing that decade's total to 240 pounds and my cumulative total to 605 pounds. Keep in mind that I was obsessed with my weight and dieting, therefore when I would gain weight back, I could quickly flush out fat, sugar, and salt with a quick loss. In a couple of weeks I could easily lose ten or fifteen pounds.

And it progressed even more

As if the addiction were not already prevalent, during the nineties the food addiction went into overdrive, that fifth gear so to speak. My all-time recorded high was in late April of 1998, 440 pounds. Most of the early nineties started out with me in the high 300's, but in 1994 I recorded my first CD called *Broadway and Stuff*. This involved putting my picture on the cover.

This project was very important to me and I wanted to look as good as possible on the front cover. I remember I weighed 345 when the picture was taken. I had probably lost about 45 pounds for that project. That now brings my total to 650 pounds lost.

The next year, 1995, I vividly remember making my second run at that same liquid diet that I went on in 1988. This time I did not quite lose 90 pounds; it was more like 80, so the new total is 730 pounds.

Lifetime high – 440 pounds

After reaching my all time high in 1998 of 440, more diets – as my pattern had established – were forthcoming. I bounced back and forth or I should say up and down another 60 pounds or so until the fall of 2002, the year Judy, my wife, died of brain cancer.

As you can imagine, it was the worst of times. I talk about the stress factor in the last section of this book. My wife in her last few months had told me that I had to take care of myself, or I was going to have a heart attack. She was right. In May of 2003, eight months after her death in September of 2002, I had triple by- pass surgery. I weighed 385 pounds at the hospital before surgery.

Ten years ago my total loss was 790 pounds. After my surgery I did gain some weight back to make one more visit to the 400-pound mark. Then…it happened…the epiphany. In April of 2005 until the publication of this book, I came close to another 210 pounds lost. My starting weight was 408 pounds. At publishing time of this book, it was about 250 pounds.

Indulge me please

This is the last set of figures you will hear. But this is important because I want you to know that even though I have done remarkably well, I have not been perfect.

I've lost approximately 190 pounds since my all time high of weighing 440. This demonstrates that even after "getting it" you cannot put it on automatic pilot. It also shows that this disease, emotional eating, is only arrested, never fully cured. Moreover I am proud to say that I am only human, but now I am a *truly happy* human. I am not perfect and never will be, but I am always making progress, feeling great and happy in my life.

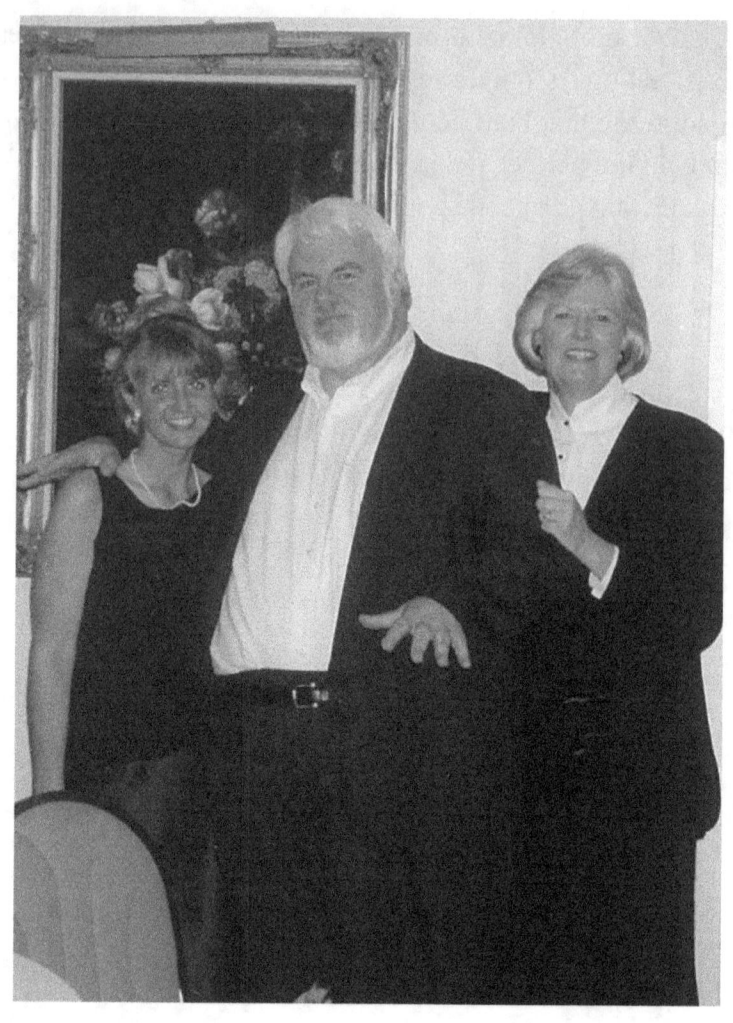

Section 2 – How I Lost The Weight

Chapter Four
How To Start On A Diet

How to start on a diet? The answer is…slowly! If that seems too simplistic, think about this. When it comes to exercise it is always recommended by everyone to start slowly and build your endurance. Slowly increase the intensity of your exercise over time. Whether you're performing aerobic (cardiovascular type exercise) or anaerobic (weight training or resistance training), "everybody" says start slowly and increase intensity to your maximum output over time. But does anybody do this with weight reduction or dieting? The answer is a resounding no! Almost no one does this. Most jump right in, wide open looking for instant results…hoping for instant gratification.

Now for a true story about starting too fast. This is one of those you had to be there, ha ha moments, spontaneous and hilarious. My physical education class in high school was scheduled for the last period of the day. After football was over, there were no planned activities in which I could engage. One day a group of us were sitting in the stands watching the tryouts for the track team. One of the participants, we'll call him Leon, was trying out for track for the first time. The event was the mile run. Some of Leon's friends had encouraged him to try and qualify for the track team by entering the mile run. After all he was naturally fast and gifted as a runner.

BANG! The gun sounded. One of the runners had bolted out of their starting stance at a pace to which we were unaccustomed. It was not a 100-meter pace, but it was somewhere between a 200 and 400 meter pace, almost wide open. We immediately erupted into laughter. By the time Leon made the first turn his stride faltered. He was gasping for breath. As he approached the second turn he started stumbling. Shortly thereafter Leon dove involuntarily into the cinder track.

I am a little ashamed to admit I rolled on the concrete floor of the stands in convulsive laughter. After all, Leon tried very hard. He had the desire to win but just did not know how to run the race. He had never been coached and was not prepared.

Remember Lincoln's quote? "If I had 60 minutes to chop down a tree, I'd spend the first 20 minutes sharpening the axe?"

As a life coach and weight loss specialist, I believe in planning and preparation. To begin dieting, like the mile run, begin slowly. The first two weeks eat exactly what you have been eating only reduce your portion size by 15% the first week, and another 15% the second week. The second week you should be eating 70% of your beginning caloric intake. This could vary with each individual however it is a good rule of thumb.

After two weeks of portion reductions of 15% each week, you may begin to concentrate on eating healthy by going on the Three Bears Diet that I have designed. In the next chapter we will discuss this diet in detail. It is simple, effective, and you will not feel deprived. It is easy to follow and it puts you on the road to getting healthy while still being able to enjoy some of your favorite foods every week.

"How To Start On A Diet" is a short chapter by design; but don't underestimate its importance. Please beware of making a "heavy" mistake… when you start a diet, start slowly.

The other thing I want to emphasize is to not deprive your body. I want you never feeling hungry. You can eat healthy building a strong immune system, while still enjoying some of your favorite foods. In the next chapter, "Eating Healthy", we will discuss your fooditude (food attitude). Next we'll talk food education, and lastly, The Three Bears Diet.

Chapter Five
Eating Healthy

Were you a member of "The Clean The Plate Club?" That term applied to most people in the United States of my generation. And if you were a part of growing up in the Southeastern United States as I did, it was a badge of honor to be in that club. Not only did I clean my plate, but there were always seconds and desserts. We called lunch dinner, and dinner, supper. And how both my maternal and paternal grandmothers could cook! Fried okra (breaded with cornmeal), sliced tomatoes, creamed corn, mashed potatoes and gravy, country fried steak, black-eyed peas and cornbread. That was for starters: but when all the extended family got together, cousins, aunts, and uncles, the smorgasbord grew to include baked ham, fried chicken, baked red snapper, and roast beef. Desserts were plentiful. My cousin and I prided ourselves in turning the crank of the ice cream freezer to produce the peach and vanilla flavors of home-made ice cream. There was an abundance of food.

Although I did not have those food courses offered me every day in my formative years, I was educated to eat like that. It was sinful to leave something on your plate. After all, there were people starving in other parts of the world. I do not mean for this to be a reflection on my parents. They did not encourage me to eat huge portions. We as growing boys were a product of the times, the post war 1950s. The I like Ike and I like food years. And my parents and their generation were products of The Great Depression where no one liked to see food wasted.

All the vegetables I ate were cooked in some type of fat. Sometimes with some sugar added and always salt. There you have those villainous ingredients, sugar, salt, and fat. Those are three things that really add to the flavor of food. There are numerous ways to substitute and reduce portions of those ingredients now. Just go to your local bookstore and browse through the food section on healthy cooking. But that was not the way it was in my childhood. And the way we ate in our childhood usually set the tone for our attitude about food, (fooditude) in later years.

Food was to be appreciated, enjoyed in large quantities, and never wasted. America's fooditude grew with my fooditude. Cheeseburgers became supersized. A bag of popcorn at the movies grew to a tub of popcorn eligible for refills. Eight-ounce sodas became thirty-two ounce sodas. Did you ever think the day would come when you would say "give me a tub of popcorn and a quart of Coke or Pepsi?" Serving sizes have doubled and tripled in the fast food industry. The supersizing of food portions served in America has led to the supersizing of our population as well.

We cannot cast the blame of increased obesity in America on any one group. We are all to blame. According to some experts, the weight gains of people in the United States can mainly be attributed to the abundance of food and the portions which we partake. Obesity will continue to grow in epidemic proportions unless we do something about it. So that brings up a question and the question is, how do we do something about it?

First it starts with the individual, like you. Do you want to do something about it? Are you ready to do something about it, and most importantly are you willing and committed to do something about it? This is where the rubber meets the road. This is where we determine your fooditude. By now you should know that is my jargon for food attitude. Most of us are not willing to change unless the burden wears too heavily on our shoulders or other parts of your body. You may have a health issue arise. You may see a picture of yourself or you may step on the scales and can't believe the number. What will it take for you to stop digging the hole? What is your bottom?

You can see from how I described my early childhood that my fooditude was that food was pleasurable, an adventure in hedonism. Get all and any kind you can get. I could only be described as a glutton. Now my attitude toward food is that it is meant to be enjoyed as healthy nourishment for our body. In working toward eating healthy your fooditude will change. Your taste buds will change and you will learn to make food taste good without piling on the sugar, salt, and fat.

Before starting on any strict regimen of a diet, you should first start eating healthy. That is another BIG SECRET I have learned about losing weight. Although our bodies can adapt to almost any kind of strict diet, it adapts much more favorably and produces better results in weight loss when our vital organs and digestive system have been receiving proper nourishment for at least thirty days. That is why for most people I recommend cutting portion sizes for the first two weeks, and then do healthy eating for four weeks or more. Then, and only then do you decide which of the diets is the right one for you. Thus another SECRET is revealed. No one diet is right for everybody. We will discuss some of them later in the book.

Before we talk about the Three Bears Diet, here is some Food Education 101. What is a calorie? Defining a calorie is a little bit like defining space. A calorie is simply a source of energy. Space you see because nothing else is there. A calorie you cannot see but you can see the results of too many of them in the form of fat. You can also see the results of having fewer of them, the reduction of fat. It takes 3,500 calories to make one pound. Each of us dependent upon our age, gender, height, weight, and frame requires a certain number of calories daily to maintain our weight. And since a calorie is a source of energy, we need to know how many of them it takes or how much energy we use daily, even if we stayed in bed all day. This is called your BMR, Basil Metabolic Rate.

To find your BMR, simply Google Basil Metabolic Rate and it will lead you to the automatic calculator. You will be asked to enter your gender, age, height, and weight. The calculator will be as accurate as possible without having a medically supervised test. What prevents it from being entirely accurate is your bone density, body frame, and muscles, in other words your individuality. However, use it as a measuring stick. Suppose your resting rate turns out to be 1800 calories per day. That is the Basil Metabolic Rate and indicates how many calories you would burn if you just remained in bed all day or did absolutely nothing. You may Google that if you wish. If you burned another 500 calories per day through exercise and regular activity, your daily calorie expenditure would be 2,300 calories. Therefore if you maintained a balanced diet of 1,300 calories, you would create a daily calorie deficit of 1,000 calories per day x seven days = 7,000 calories per week. Remember that it takes 3,500 calories to make a pound. Theoretically, you should lose two pounds that week. If you choose to follow that 1,300-calorie diet, what is it? What foods make up my 1,300 calories?

What cals should be my pals? Choose your calories like you choose your friends. You want a friend that will listen to you in time of need and encourage you to pursue your interests and goals. You would also like a friend to help you to maintain your emotional health and positive attitude. The food of which you partake should do that as well. Good food should satisfy your hunger. Nutritionally sound foods proportionally distributed will not only provide a healthy body, but also a healthy mind. The following is a discussion of the food groups.

CARBOHYDRATES

Carbohydrate next to water is consumed more than any other food source in the world. It is the main fuel source for the body. One gram of carbohydrate contains four calories. Glucose, the simplest carbohydrate is a must for brain cells, red blood cells, and is a main energy source for strenuous exercise (source *The New Glucose Revolution*, page 11). There are three kinds of carbs; sugars, starches, and fiber. Milk, honey, brown sugar, table sugar, molasses, sugar, yogurt and fruit are sugars. Fruit, milk, and yogurt are natural sugars. Starches are made up from sugar units. They are slower to digest and provide sustained energy. They can be found in grains, rice, pasta, beans/lentils, bread and cereal. There are also starchy vegetables such as potatoes, peas, and corn.

What is fiber? Fiber is the part of the plant that cannot be fully digested by the body. Fiber plays a crucial role in preventing the bacteria in our body from becoming toxic buildup. Not only does fiber give texture and volume to food; additionally it is a wonderful cleansing system for our body, promoting regularity. Fiber is found in fruits, vegetables, and whole grains. When choosing whole grains, be sure they are unprocessed or limited processed whole grains such as 100% wheat bread, brown rice, and old fashioned regular oatmeal. Refining of the grains removes the fiber you need as well as some important nutrients.

THE GLYCEMIC INDEX

The glycemic index measures how each food impacts our blood sugar or blood glucose. High glycemic carbohydrates send more sugar in the bloodstream. The hormone insulin, which is created by the pancreas, carries this glucose to our muscles and cells. If there is too much sugar in our blood the pancreas is overworked and this could cause diabetes. With lower glycemic carbs we stay full longer because they are digested more slowly. Our diet can control how much sugar we have in our blood. A diabetic sometimes needs insulin shots to help carry the extra glucose to the muscles and cells. Some organizations such as The American Diabetes Association do not deem the glycemic index very practical because it measures each food singularly while foods are usually ingested with other foods as part of a meal. This is where you use common sense. Honey is very high on the glycemic index: therefore, you would not want to eat it in large quantities. But a little bit of honey is probably good for you especially after a workout with weights as it sends glucose quickly to the muscles.

PROTEIN

Protein, like carbohydrates, has four calories per gram. One of the jobs of protein is to maintain muscle and some of the vital organs like the heart, kidneys, and lungs. Protein helps create antibodies that fight infection along with helping to form red blood cells. Protein is like a string of pearls, each representing an amino acid. There are twenty of these, nine of which are called essential, meaning the body can't make them: therefore they must be supplied by food. The other amino acids are called non-essential because your body can synthesize them. High quality food sources such as meat, fish, dairy, and eggs should meet the essential protein requirements your body needs.

FATS

Where carbs and protein have four calories per gram, fats have nine. Fat is what gives texture and flavor to a lot of the foods we eat. Fat is stored in fat cells which help preserve body heat. Fat is a source of energy, like carbohydrates. There are basically three kinds of fats: saturated fats, unsaturated fats, and trans fats. Saturated fats are solid at room temperature. They can raise your blood cholesterol level so they really need to be eaten in moderation. Some examples of saturated fats would be cheese, whole milk, ice cream, butter, lard, and high fat meats such as heavily marbled beef, spareribs, and sausage. Eating some saturated fats is ok. Just do it in small portions and infrequently.

Fats to be eaten even less frequently would be in cookies, donuts, shortening, cakes, crackers, and French fries. These are called trans fats and they will also raise cholesterol levels. Unsaturated fats are the good guys. They are liquid at room temperatures and actually help to lower bad cholesterol (LDL). They may also help to raise the good cholesterol (HDL).

There is polyunsaturated fat such as corn oil, sunflower oil, fish oil, safflower oil, and walnuts. There are monounsaturated fats such as extra virgin olive oil, canola oil, peanut oil, avocados, almonds, and most other nuts. Once again I must caution you on your portions. Four tablespoons of olive oil is 480 calories. Remember fat has 9 calories per gram.

There you have your basic food education. You need a balanced food plan of these different food groups to eat healthy. I have developed an eating plan that will energize you and help develop your immune system. I call it the Three Bears Diet.

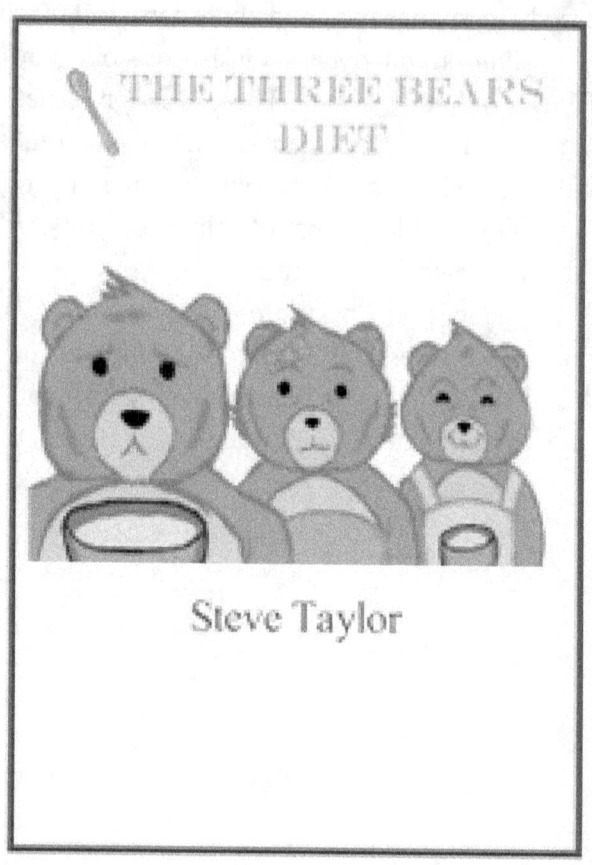

THE THREE BEARS DIET

Steve Taylor

The Three Bears Diet

Once upon a time there was a young girl named Goldylocks or was it Goldilocks? Well never mind about that, I am probably dating myself with that reference. However, she did meet up with these three bears by breaking into their house and observing their personal dinnerware, namely their porridge bowls. There was that tiny bowl for the Baby bear, the medium size bowl for the Mama bear, and the large bowl for the Papa bear. This just goes to show you that animals do a pretty good job of portion control. Take my seventeen-year-old toy poodle, "Bernie". You can put a lot of food before him, but he will take only what he needs most of the time. This is called practicing portion control. Unfortunately, we of the human species do not do such a good job of portioning what we eat.

Earlier in this chapter, I talk about how the preponderance of food in America has made us fat. Learning portion control and how to implement it provides us an opportunity to help reduce our waistline. The Three Bears Diet requires that you measure your food intake based upon the size of the palm of your hand, or fist, in the case of food shaped like a potato. Each serving of food therefore is about the size of the palm of your hand. You don't have to weigh it. Just look at your hand.

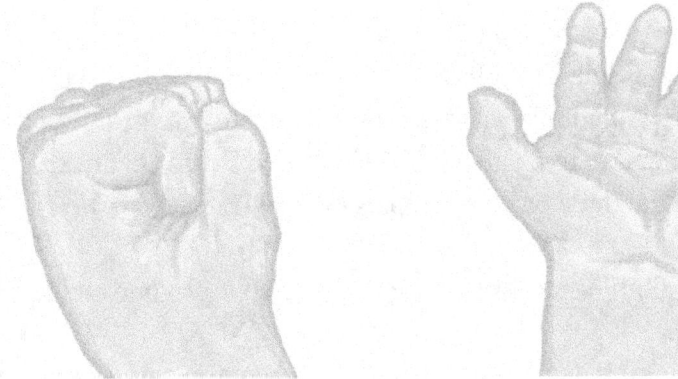

Portion control:
Use the size of your fist or the palm of your hand

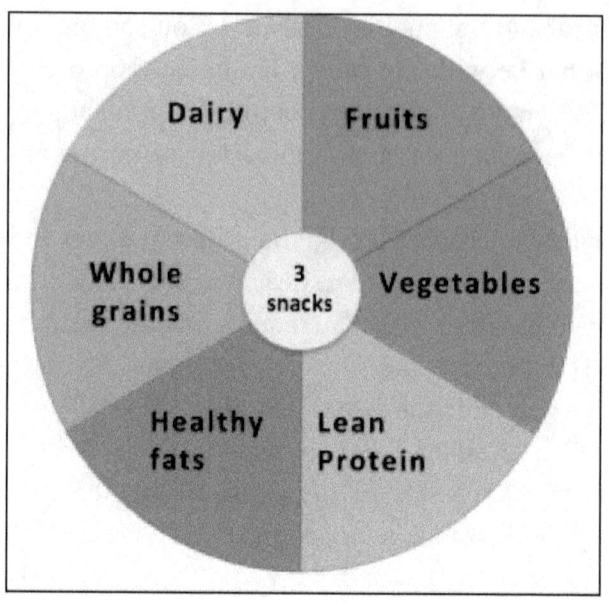

Three servings daily from the six food groups

The Three Bears Diet also suggests that you have three servings daily, in the first phase of the diet, from each of six food groups. These include fruits, vegetables, lean protein, healthy fats, whole grains, and dairy. This makes The Three Bears Diet healthy.

Here are the three basic principles of The Three Bear Diet:

(1) It is simple, healthy, and helps you control your intake of food.

(2) It provides for three snacks per day and even allows you flexibility to eat your favorite foods.

(3) It can easily be amended to become two other diets, Zone or Atkins.

Now lets look at each of these principles a little closer.

The first one is pretty self-explanatory. By controlling your intake of food, you will lose weight and if a program is simple and easy to follow, you'll stay on it longer and reach your goal faster. Of course you also want to stay healthy while you're doing it.

The second principle is related to snacking. You are allowed three of your favorite foods three times per week in one of those snacks. You can have anything you want as long as it does not exceed 100 calories. Three snacks per day, for seven days equals 21 snacks per week. Eighteen of those snacks should be healthy. I recommend a small portion of fruit and low-fat cottage cheese or Okios non-fat Greek Yogurt. I have found that it expedites weight loss when you combine a protein with a carbohydrate.

The other three of those snacks can be anything, even though it may not rank so high on the nutrition chart. This could be a big slice of pizza or a partial cup of the richest ice cream you can find. It is difficult to keep these type of snacks under 100 calories, so okay fudge a little; but do watch your portions. Allowing yourself these "anything goes" snacks keeps you from feeling deprived. Instead of the three weekly "anything goes" snacks, I eat one meal per week of anything I want. I usually do this by dining out for the evening meal on the weekends. Even though I order what I want, I do not pig out. I piglet out. You know the difference; but I will gladly give you an illustration.

If you were to choose a fast food restaurant, let's say a Wendy's, I might order a single with cheese, small order of fries and a regular Frosty. I would not order a triple with cheese, large fries, and a large frosty. It is about portion control. The Three Bears Diet allows us to portion our food while not depriving ourselves.

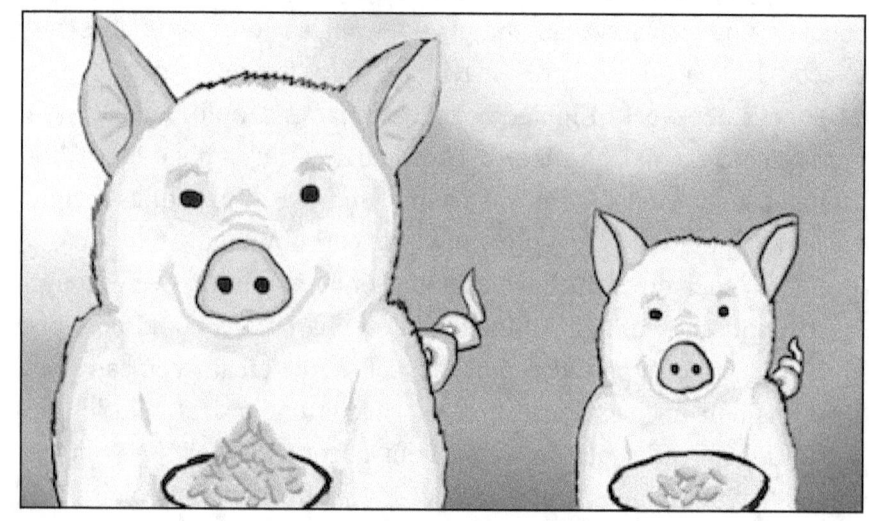

Don't pig out...piglet out!

The third principle concerns altering The Three Bears Diet to look more like either the Zone Diet or Atkins. Both can accelerate your weight loss. The first way we can change the diet is to take away, as seen below, the whole grain servings, the dairy servings, and the snacks. You now have what is very close to the Zone Diet. I very much like this diet. You can lose weight at a healthy but good pace, faster than you can on The Three Bears Diet.

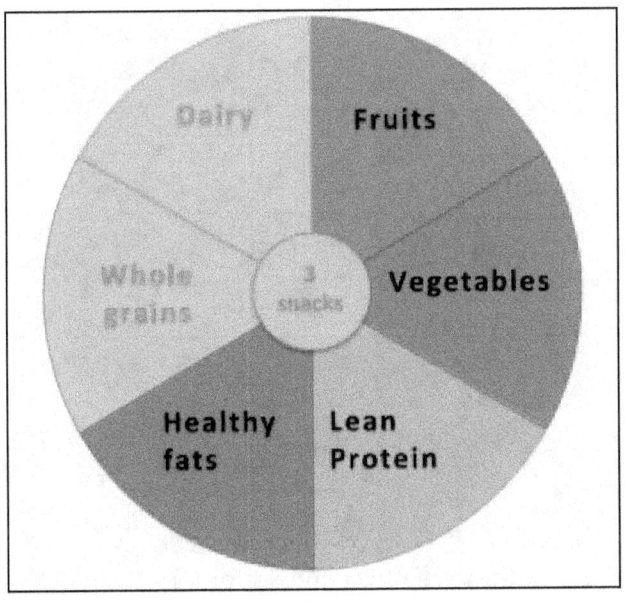

The Three Bears to Zone Diet

Another way to amend the diet is to eliminate all of the servings of dairy, whole grains, snacks, and fruits. You now have the Atkins diet.

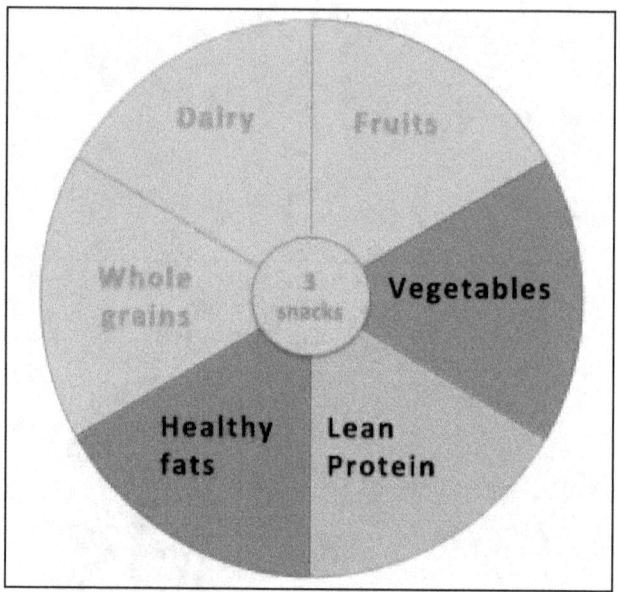

The Three Bears to Atkins Diet

With both of these changes you are eliminating carbohydrates, which are found in those food groups. I prefer the Zone over the Atkins because I can have fruit. I have found the rapidity of the weight loss to be about the same, with Atkins having a little bit of an edge. However, that is only for me. You will have to see what works best for you.

You may still have a couple of snacks; but I would make it fruit and low-fat cottage cheese. You may still have your one meal a week of anything of your choosing, as long as you just piglet out.

With Atkins you can have any kind of fat including cheese, saturated fats in prime cuts of beef, and egg yolks. With the Zone Diet you are encouraged to eat only healthy fats such as extra virgin olive oil, walnuts, and almonds. I also take an Omega 3 fish oil.

As you can see The Three Bears Diet is flexible and convertible into two other diets that probably will make you lose weight faster. It certainly will not hurt you to do these other diets as long as you are healthy and your physician approves. My personal experience was that I did occasionally feel a little hunger on both of these programs. Having one piece of bread would usually cure that.

As I've mentioned before, I do recommend that you start dieting slowly, eating a combination of all the healthy food groups. This not only will establish a healthy eating lifestyle for you; moreover, it will make you healthy.

Start first with the Three Bears Diet. Establish healthy eating but don't deprive. Have your three weekly snacks of anything you want or your one meal of anything you want. Then stick to the other food choices I have outlined for you. Here is what the Mama Bear portions and menu may look like.

The Three Bears Diet: Mama Bear Portions

Breakfast
½ grapefruit
½ cup regular oatmeal
1 slice turkey bacon

OR

½ cup low fat small curd cottage cheese with sliced apples

1 slice of reduced sugar 100% whole wheat bread
   OR

2 eggs scrambled, with one yolk removed

½ cantaloupe

1 slice of reduced sugar 100% whole wheat bread

Lunch

1 piece of fruit

1 salad with all color veggies, a sprinkle of mozzarella cheese, one teaspoon of extra virgin olive oil and either lemon juice or vinegar
   OR

Spinach (boiled or steamed), collards, broccoli, or squash

Lean protein – chicken, fish, or turkey – a handful cooked as you wish, but not fried

Dinner

Same as lunch, but vary the ingredients you use

Snacks

Yogurt, preferably Greek, with fruit

A handful of walnuts or almonds, twice a day

Here is a review of authorized foods in each category:

Authorized Foods by Category

Lean Protein

93% lean ground beef, chicken breasts or strips, turkey breasts, white fish, salmon, tuna, shrimp, tilapia fillets, low fat cottage cheese, egg whites, and buffalo. Other sources of lean protein are: beans, nuts, legumes, and grains.

Fruit
Any fruits with the exception of avocados

Vegetables
Squash, cucumbers, spinach, kale, collard and turnip greens, and any other low calorie low carb vegetables. Limit starchy vegetables such as peas, corn, and baked potatoes (substitute sweet potatoes)

Dairy
Low fat and low sugar yogurt, nonfat milk, and nonfat cheese

Healthy Fats
Extra virgin olive oil (it is important to use one tablespoon daily) then choose two others from avocados, almonds, or walnuts, or any healthy fat in the food education section.

Whole Grains
100% whole-wheat products with reduced sugar: one slice is a Papa Bear serving; ½ slice is for Mama Bear. Other authorized products are old-fashioned oatmeal and high fiber cereals with low carbs, fat, and sugar content

Snacks
Anything healthy at 100 calories or less

Conclusion
Stay on the Three Bears Diet for at least four weeks. You should lose one to two pounds per week and should never be hungry. Then if that rate of weight loss is too slow for you, convert it to Atkins or The Zone or your favorite weight loss program that I discuss throughout the book.

NOW would be the best time to get started. You may contact me at www.stevetaylormyownweigh.com to set up a free 20-minute consult via phone.

The Three Bears Diet is very simple and it is healthy. This is what I did to begin my journey of eating healthy. After being on this diet for four weeks, you can then go on any diet you choose. Your body's engine will be working so much better after you have invested in this new fuel for it. It will show its appreciation for you by making you feel better in every respect. Since you now probably have a greater resistance to illness in the way of a healthier body, you can now probably challenge yourself a little more if you wish for the purpose of losing weight faster. It is better to have patience; but believe me I'm one of you I know how it is. You want to get the weight off now.

This next chapter will be a critique and my personal opinion of some of the best-known diets of the ones I have been on.

Chapter Six
A Diets Critique

Over the last forty or fifty years these are some of the diets of which I was a participant. The Mayo Clinic Diet, The South Beach Diet, The Mediterranean Diet, The T Factor Diet, The Atkins Diet, The HCG Diet, LA Weight Loss, Weight Watchers, The Eating For Life Diet, Medifast Diet (nothing but liquid supplement), The Three Day Diet, Numerous variations of counting calories, Jenny Craig, Nutrisystem, Ediets, and Sugar Busters. Is this a good stopping point? I could probably think of at least a dozen more; but hopefully I have made my point.

There is so much information out there about the right way to diet, each claiming to be the best approach and the end all answer to dieting. The T Factor diet restricted fats and you counted fat grams, initially restricting them to 20 per day. You don't hear much about it anymore, but there are variations of fat restrictive diets out there.

Then there is The Atkins Diet. It restricts carbohydrates to 20 grams per day and most of the carbohydrates you get from vegetables.

Medifast, since I did it has been modified, but at the time it consisted of drinking a liquid where you only get about 500 calories per day.

The HCG Diet only allows you 500 calories per day, plus you take drops or injections of Human Chorionic Gonadotropin, a hormone secreted by a woman during pregnancy to deliver fat to the fetus. The idea is that the fat gives you enough energy to compensate for the low caloric intake. Most experts say that you lose weight on this diet not because of the HCG but the low caloric intake. You can lose up to 10 pounds per week on this and the claim is that is fat only, no muscle.

The diet industry is growing because people are getting fatter. Mix a buck in there and see how many diets and claims we can come up with. There is a song from *Fiddler On The Roof,* one of the greatest musicals of all time, called "If I Were A Rich Man." There is a line in that song that says, "If you're rich they think you really know."

If you have the title of Dr. in front of your name or you have been on Oprah or Dr. Oz people think you really know. Folks, I am here to tell you, they don't really know. I truly respect and admire Oprah and Dr. Oz and most people in the medical profession. I am just cautioning you to be careful. The diet industry is a huge business. All of these diets work but which one is healthy? Can you keep the weight off?

Here is what I think and what I did. I looked to find what region of the world people lived the longest and what their diet was. It is around the Mediterranean Sea where they eat healthy fats such as extra virgin olive oil, and nuts, a lot of vegetables and fruit, fresh of course, and small quantities of meat, and whole grains. Thus, the Mediterranean diet or my version, The Three Bears Diet.

I also talked to body builders who had to lose fat and have their bodies in tiptop shape for competition and asked them how they did it. Every man and woman told me the same thing. They ate a balanced diet but restricted fats and carbs and ate about six times per day. Most all took supplements especially Omega 3's.

Dr. Barry Sears is the author of the Zone diet, which basically says that inflammation causes storage of extra fat in fat cells. Dr. Sears says put lean meat the size of your palm on about one third of your plate and two thirds should be fruits and vegetables. Dr. Sears emphasizes the importance of the healthy fats, especially fish oil. This diet restricts carbs and unhealthy fats and emphasizes healthy fats. This is what I truly have come to believe over the years, you should do. As I mentioned before I like the Zone diet very much and I use it frequently. I believe it to be much like The Mediterranean diet and it is simple to follow. I have plenty of energy on it; and it is highly effective for weight loss.

Weight Watchers and Jenny Craig, two really good programs emphasize fruits and vegetables as well. In fact, anything that is produced naturally and preferably organically or grown by The God of your choosing is good for you.

No one diet is right for everyone but the Zone Diet and the Mediterranean Diet are both great. I also recommend Weight Watchers to a lot of people. You have accountability by attending meetings and weighing every week. You receive food education from your group and group leader. Group leaders are only chosen from people who have lost weight and maintained their weight loss on Weight Watchers. They are also well trained in food education.

Jenny Craig is owned by Nestles, a big company that makes lean cuisine. They have a counselor who calls you once a week to discuss your progress or lack thereof, and every two weeks deliver you pre-prepared food. Most of the food is pretty good, much of it fresh frozen. If you do not like to cook or lack the time this is a great program.

Nutrisystem is also a good program that I think has made some strides recently in improving the quality of their food. They are not quite there with Jenny Craig in quality but very close. Although counseling is available online, it is not as personalized as Jenny Craig. However, there is one big advantage that Nutrisystem has, it is less expensive. Which one is better? It is a toss-up.

Remember I said body builders know how to lose weight and stay healthy. Bill Phillips of *Body For Life* fame has a program called "The Eating For Life method." It restricts carbs and fats, except for healthy ones and is extremely easy to follow. I highly recommend you read this book *Body for Life*. In the early 2000s it was on the New York Times non-fiction bestseller list for many months. Bill has a company called EAS supplements and has trained many world-class athletes. I believe what Bill Phillips says.

Body for Life is one of a few books that I wish everyone would read that is seeking the truth about diet and exercise.

One of the other books is called *The Worlds Healthiest Foods: Essential Guide for the Healthiest Way of Eating*. George Mateljan is the author. It could not be more credible or more thorough. It rates each of the food groups' healthiest foods and tells you how to select and cook them. In my opinion, no one can touch George Mateljan for knowledge and honesty. In fact if you like to cook, his diet, which is basically the Mediterranean Diet, would be my number one choice. My wife and I just don't like to cook, even though most of George's recipes take 10 minutes or less.

I currently adhere closely to my creation, The Three Bears Diet, with an emphasis on watching fat grams while making sure I am eating my healthy fats. Since I am healthy, I have built my immune system. I have only had two minor colds in the last four or five years. And because of my normally good eating habits, I am still able to enjoy a stadium hotdog at football games and an occasional favorite treat such as ice cream and chocolate syrup.

THE DEVIL IN DISGUISE, SEVERELY RESTRICTED CARBOHYDRATE DIETS

As you may imagine after reading my story, over the years through suffering and experimentation resulting in resounding success, I have developed some pretty strong opinions of the diet industry and the different kinds of diets I have tried. That is why I feel it is necessary to address this issue of the diet revolution that probably started with the Atkins diet. Now, almost every diet that has evolved over the last few years is some form of very low carb diet, like South Beach, Wheat Belly, Paleo, Duchan, and the list goes on.

Here is what happened to me every time I tried one of those diets. I would lose a lot of weight rapidly during the initial stages of the diet but then I would quickly hit a plateau. Even though I was eating a severely restricted number of calories, I was barely losing weight. Additionally my training at the gym was suffering. I simply did not have enough energy to exercise the way I wanted to. Why didn't I have enough energy? The answer is I was depleting my body of its main fuel source, carbohydrates. Allow me to quote veteran fitness industry guru and bestselling author Tom Venuto. On page 6 in his new book, *Burn The Fat Feed The Muscle,* he states, "reduce your carbohydrates too much and your energy level takes a dive." I strongly encourage you to read *Burn The Fat Feed The Muscle* by Tom Venuto.

For my next expert witness regarding this reduced carb myth, I call Dr. Martin Katahn, Ph.D., author of New York Times bestseller list (23 weeks), *The T-Factor Diet*. At its publication in 1989, Dr. Katahn was director of the Vanderbilt Weight Management program at Vanderbilt University. Most of the carbohydrates we eat are transformed to a form of sugar called glycogen. In the section called "How the Body Stores Fuel" on pages sixteen and seventeen, *The T-Factor Diet*, here is what Dr. Katahn says about glycogen:

"The glycogen is stored in a solution of water, about 3 to 4 parts water to 1 part glycogen. For every 500 calories of glycogen stored, enough water is combined with it to equal one pound of body weight. Thus whenever you increase or decrease just 500 calories of your glycogen stores, you gain or lose a pound of body weight, but it's mostly water. Part of the daily weight fluctuation we all experience is due to variation in our carbohydrate intake, as well as our salt intake, which also influences water retention.

Quick weight loss diets that cut out carbohydrates in the diet capitalize on glycogen depletion, to give you a spurious weight loss; the water weight is regained immediately upon any increase in calorie consumption.

Fast weight loss diets that cut back on the carbohydrates count on the water loss that accompanies the depletion of your glycogen stores to make the diets more attractive and encourage you to try them."

These are quotes from a renowned expert from one of our Country's finest Universities. I will not go into the comparison of how the body stores fat, but I encourage you to purchase and read this book.

There you have it...an opinion from an exercise expert, a doctor who originated the T-Factor Diet, and me, a guy who has actually tried all this stuff and all that goes with it like the lipotropic injections, fat burners, etc.

I hope that you do not think this trashing of low carb diets hypocritical of me. After all, wasn't I the one that said just a few pages back you could easily convert The Three Bears Diet to Atkins? The fact is that some people, mainly men, feel like they have to eat lots of meat and fat like blue cheese, but they can do without carbs. Although I really disagree with this, I support anyone in his or her efforts to lose weight. I would never say my way is the only way to lose weight. That is actually what the title of the book means, My OWN Weigh. The OWN is emphasized because in order to be successful, you have to "own" what you are doing. That translates to say you have to believe in what you are doing and it has to be your idea.

By now you should have some questions. If you do, I hope you find it in the next section. If not email me, at: steve@stevetaylormyownweigh.com and I will respond.

Chapter Seven
Frequently Asked Questions

People ask me the same questions over and over. In an attempt to summarize them and put them in a single spot for reference, I've compiled a list so I can answer them for you all at once. Here they are:

1) How much should I weigh?

That is up to you and your doctor to decide, not the insurance charts. For example I am 6' 3" with a big frame. My blood levels and blood pressure are good. This tells a lot about your health. I have had two very good Internal Medicine Docs with a lot of experience say 240 and 250 respectively for my weight. Some of the charts show my ideal weight at just over 200 pounds. Sorry, I am not going there. I like to stay close to 250.

2) How should I give my weight, stripped or with clothes on?

Weigh in the morning in your underwear shorts after voiding. That was how I was told to weigh when I was in the hospital. I would suggest we all have some fun and give our height with our shoes on and weight with our clothes off.

3) What is a safe rate to lose weight?

You can lose up to 1% of your starting weight per week. If your starting weight is 300 that would be three pounds per week. Most experts recommend one to two pounds per week. They say that losing more than that means you are losing muscle, which slows your metabolism.

4) Should I exercise while losing weight?

You should exercise while losing weight with aerobic and anaerobic exercise, which will be covered in the chapter on exercise.

5) How much of losing weight is exercise and how much is your diet?

Your diet accounts for about 80% of your success. Exercise accounts for about 20%. But oh how important that 20% is.

6) Will I get hungry and feel deprived?

If you read the chapters on How To Start On A Diet and Eating Healthy and implement my program, you will not get hungry.

7) Should I drink a lot of water?

Yes, you should drink a lot of water, 6 to 8 eight ounce glasses per day no matter what kind of diet you are on. The water should be drunk in addition to your other liquids like coffee or tea.

8) Can I eat out?

Of course you can eat out. I do it all the time. Prepare your cooked vegetables that you eat at home by steaming and not cooking with fat. My wife and I steam a lot of broccoli and spinach and refrigerate them. When we are eating out we eat raw veggies (salads) or seasonal fresh cooked in olive oil.

9) Will my taste for food change and will I lose my cravings for the bad stuff?

Your taste for food and your food attitude will change. I was a steak and loaded baked potato man for years. I still like steak and eat it occasionally. I always searched for the really prime cuts, that corn fed beef that give it flavor. I know now that is saturated fat and I did not like having my chest sawed open, (triple by-pass). To satisfy your sweet tooth, eating fruit with natural sugar will help absolve that craving. I am not saying it will entirely disappear but when you are eating healthy, you will be amazed at how your food tastes will change. And here is the whole point in going through what I have asked you to do. You will be a new person with a new attitude. What would be the point in doing all of this if you were still addicted to food, got hungry, and craved certain foods? You would be miserable. So remember…if you suffer, there's hope for you and we are going to end the suffering!

10) If I do this on my own without attending Weight Watchers or Jenny Craig, can I get support?

There is a website called sparkpeople.com that will give you support. Also, I am a weight loss coach, counselor, and mentor. If you are interested in my services, go to stevetaylormyownweigh.com for more info.

11) What about supplements, do I need them?

I think you do need some supplementation. There is a warehouse distributor called All Star Health in California where I buy Lean Body Shake. This is a delicious tasting supplement by Lee Labrada. Myoplex by EAS, is a Bill Phillips product and any of those are good. Frankly, I cannot tell you which products are best.

As this revision goes to publication, a new controversy over supplements has just emerged. The studies have shown that if you eat the right foods you do not need supplements. Duh…that is why they are called supplements. I do not always eat the right foods. Here is what I take most of the time. There is a company called The Synergy Company out of Moab, Utah. There is a wellness pack my wife and I use consisting of multi-vitamins and a super food, both organically grown. We both agree this is the best supplement we have ever taken. We can immediately tell the difference in our energy levels, and it provides excellent cleaning capability for our bodies. Their website is TheSynergyCompany.com. Their phone number is 800-723-0277.

As always, it is good to check with your doctor before taking any supplements.

12) Do fat burners or any of those products I see advertised work to speed metabolism and accentuate weight loss?

It has been my experience and the opinion of most experts that they do not. I believe that healthy fats are your best fat burners. I don't know how you would ever tell for sure who had the best products but I would recommend doing your own research and experimentation. I buy Omega 3 from Carlson. It is liquid and comes in a couple of flavors. Lemon is my choice. A spoonful per day seems to keep my skin from becoming red and dry. Check the prices on Amazon.com or Vitacost.com. It is sold in Target, but you can save money buying it on line.

13) Does diet pop or soda have an impact on weight loss?

As you probably are aware, there is quite a debate on this. I do not think a couple of diet drinks per day will affect your weight loss. There are several well- known weight loss people that are against them. In losing 180 pounds, they did not seem to affect me.

14) Are artificial sweeteners good for you and do they help or hinder weight loss?

Here we go again, another debate. They are good for you only in the sense that they have no calories. The general consensus now is that Stevia or Truvia is what you should use. That is what I use at home. They are more expensive than Splenda, which is most often found in restaurants. A little bit of old regular processed sugar every once in a while won't hurt you.

15) Do you recommend more than three meals a day and if so when should they be eaten?

In order for you to boost your metabolism, I recommend eating at least five times per day. Notice in The Three Bears Diet, three snacks per day are allowed making for a total of eating six times per day. Have a mid-morning, mid-afternoon, and an early evening snack if desired.

16) What is your opinion on processed foods and their impact on weight?

Every time food is heated or processed some nutrients are lost. Buy organic until your pocketbook becomes uncomfortable. If you are eating healthy and your body is nutritionally sound, and you are exercising, you will lose weight naturally without feeling deprived or suffering.

17) Are you familiar with Garcinia Cambogia and other weight loss supplements such as Green Coffee Beans? Do they work or are they just like all the other fat burners?

Although I have not tried Garcinia Cambogia, I have tried several different green teas along with the Raspberry Ketones. I wish I had my money back! I repeat the only good fat burners are healthy fats in moderation!!!!

18) If you are against low-carb diets and all these weight loss supplements, why are they out there? Many of them have loads of testimonials.

THANKYOU! You have given me a chance to bloviate. My business background is in advertising and marketing. People respond emotionally in making purchases. We humans, by nature, are always looking for an easier softer way or that special deal. Sellers know this and appeal to you accordingly. Look at a huge sector of our economy, the automobile industry. The commercials you see on television show file footage of the excitement of driving their car. Whether it is sliding in after a spin on the road as in fun to drive or a happy family enjoying their SUV, they are appealing to your emotions. Food companies respond to customer demands. Since the rage for the last few years has been low carb, and more low carb, those are the products offered to the consumer. The whole idea of this book is to tell how I did it, and tell what I perceive to be the truth about the diet industry.

Chapter Eight
Exercise

Wow! Like dieting, volumes and volumes have been written on this subject. What do I do? Can't this stuff become addictive? Yeah, it can become addictive; but in all likelihood it won't. Even if it does, isn't that better than being 200 pounds overweight? My daughter was at one time very heavy. She now has run four or five marathons. By her own admission, she may be addicted to exercise. She loves the way it makes her feel, and she looks great! It seems this weight thing involves genetics.

To begin an exercise program, there are two places you can start, outside, or in the gym. We are going to talk about two different kinds of exercise. I think you should consider doing them both. This is what I did which greatly enhanced my physical and mental health.

The first is aerobic exercise. Aerobic literally means with air. It is also referred to as cardio as it stimulates the very important muscle, the heart. Most all of us have done aerobic exercise at one time or another like walking, running, swimming, cycling, tennis, or any kind of game like volleyball, etc. that requires movement and using a lot of air. Aerobics improve skin color, circulation, and slows down the aging process. How much aerobic exercise you should do and how deep into it you want to get depends on you.

If you have not exercised in a long time and are grossly overweight, start walking ten minutes per day. The second week, make it 12 minutes per day, the third 15, and the fourth 20. By the end of 6 weeks you should be walking 30 minutes per day for five days. There is no need to ever go above that unless you just want to, just work on quickening the pace. In Bill Phillips' book *Body For Life,* he talks about how long you should exercise aerobically and anaerobically. There is no need to build up to spend all day exercising for optimum health. What about the rest of your life? When you walk it is best to do it first thing in the morning before eating. Your metabolism will increase better this way. "Scientific studies indicate that fat is burned much faster- up to 300% faster when you exercise in the morning as opposed to doing the same exercise in the afternoon." Bill Phillips, *Body For Life*, page 65.

The illustration I used about Leon's first mile run in the chapter on How To Start On A Diet certainly applies to exercise as well. Start slowly and you will finish big. I have already given you the biggest secret of cardio, thanks to Bill Phillips. Do it in the morning. Get started. Pick out something you like and do it at your own pace. Buy a spiral notebook and keep records. I have them everywhere. Thank you, Dollar General!

Anaerobic exercise consists of resistance and weight training. Over the years weight training has become better understood and the true benefits of it have been discovered. There are those who think it is just as important as cardiovascular exercise. It really can prepare us more to be before we are ready not to be, nothing like a little Shakespeare. Weight training builds muscle that increases metabolism that helps eliminate fat.

It also makes for stronger bones, a critical issue with senior citizens. Anaerobic exercise decreases the chance of osteoporosis occurring. If you are not a senior citizen your goal should be to become one and when you do to have stronger bones. The best advice I could give anyone that is embarking on a weight training program is to join a gym before you invest in equipment. Find one with a good reputation that will offer you some free training sessions initially with a trainer. Get a commitment from them to educate you, particularly with free weights. I could recommend some exercises; however, I am not a personal trainer. There are many dedicated, well-educated, good ones out there with a desire to help people.

If you do not have access to a gym, start with dumbbells only and a weight bench, no barbells. Read *Body For Life* by Bill Phillips. Again, I also highly recommend the book *Burn The Fat Feed The Muscle* by Tom Venuto. Venuto is a twenty-five year veteran of the fitness industry and bestselling author. Or look on the Internet for beginner exercises. If you are not a beginner you know what to do. I am living proof that starting an exercise program like I have described along with a proper diet will make you lose weight, transform your body and your life. Get started. And by the way that is what the last chapter is about, getting started.

Section 3 – Psychology of Overeating

Chapter Nine
Emotional Eating

The National Institute of Health estimates that about 98% or better of persons gain their weight back after dieting. Why is this happening? The answer lies in the big secret that I am going to share with you, EMOTIONAL EATING. Emotional eating was totally ignored for years in weight loss. No diets or food plans addressed it. Recently (within the last few years) some of the major weight loss programs such as Weight Watchers and Jenny Craig have addressed the issue but they don't go into emotional eating in depth. These are both really good programs, I have done them both, and I am sure they have valid reasons for not addressing them more, maybe fear of lawsuits. Who knows? This book will put emotional eating under a microscope and I will show you how I arrested it. EMOTIONAL EATING must be arrested for long-term success!

Get ready to embark for we are addressing the root of the problem. If you are willing to implement the principles in this book, your transformation will amaze you.

Okay, so the cat's out of the bag. We have identified a problem that affects most people who are obese (20% or more overweight) or morbidly obese (100 pounds or more overweight). The culprit is called, emotional eating, it's the reason we cannot keep from regaining that weight back we lost after dieting. So what is emotional eating? Is it some form of eating disorder or addiction? Yes, it is.

Most of what I have learned about eating disorders came from practical, real life experiences and attendance at an eating disorder clinic in the mid-eighties. Here is a description of an eating disorder.

The taste of food and the process of eating it, like chewing and swallowing create intense sensations. These sensations are so powerful that they can remove and replace some other unpleasant feeling that the person can be experiencing. Food becomes the enabler and serves as a coping mechanism for dealing with emotional pain. Therefore, instead of eating to serve our body's needs, we are eating to prevent the emotional agony we may be enduring. When we repeatedly eat to deal with emotional pain, we eventually and unconsciously respond automatically. Thus we cross the line. We are now addicted. We have an eating disorder. I am a recovering food addict. Most of my life I have dealt with emotional pain through food. Pain is pain. And sometimes, emotional pain can be greater than physical pain. It leads to stress – and stress is a killer.

I'm convinced that stress was the catalyst for my heart attack and eventual triple bypass surgery. My unhealthy lifestyle certainly was a major contributor. I had the stress of a business to run, and had just lost my wife after a nine-month battle with brain cancer. I was drinking too much alcohol, overeating and smoking. I did some weight training but not much cardio. It is no surprise that I had the heart attack. I know stress and what it can do to you.

There are all kinds of things that cause emotional pain. Emotional pain usually is a derivative of a loss of one's self. Loss of one's self usually comes from the loss of another person, such as a death, or a break-up in a relationship, or a conflict with another person. We know who we are by the nature of our relationships with other people. When we lose that we simply lose part of ourselves. Then some of us turn to eating to push out the pain.

All this brings up a question. If emotional pain is so devastating and unhealthy and causes overeating, how do we deal with it? As I promised you earlier, if you suffer, there is hope for you. Help is on the way. Here is how I dealt with it.

There are seven principles that must be followed in order to conquer emotional eating. I am going to take you through them in detail in the next two chapters, but here they are so you can familiarize yourself with all seven of them:

Surrender:

1. Admit to yourself that the way you view and ingest food is out of control, and that you cannot manage your eating on a consistent basis, especially after dieting.
2. Come to the realization that an ultimate authority of spiritual magnitude will be needed to help you control your emotional eating.
3. Have belief that this ultimate authority of spiritual magnitude (the God of your choosing) could arrest your emotional eating and become willing to turn this burden over to him.

Brain Flush:

4. Make a list of all your resentments against people, places, or institutions, and make a list of all of your fears.
5. Discuss these in detail with another person who is a qualified professional or someone you completely trust.
6. Make a list of people that you may have harmed.
7. Seek out these people and apologize and make amends whenever possible.

Once you have gone through these seven principles, you will be well on your way to recovery from emotional eating. Continue to follow along as I help you through the process in the next chapters.

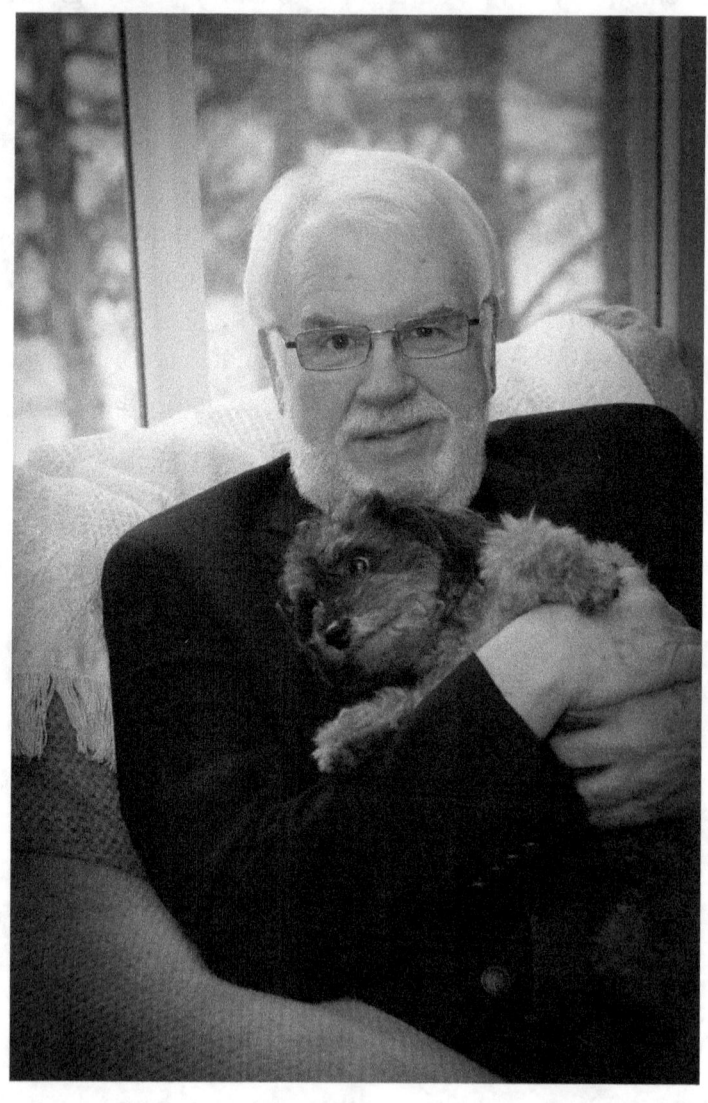

Chapter Ten
Surrender

The first action required to expel the obsession of emotional eating is to surrender. No way you say! I'm not giving up. I'll never meet my weight loss goal of permanence by giving up. What do you want me to do, admit defeat and remain obese? Of course not, here is why surrendering is not giving up. The three phases of the surrender process are: 1) Admit to yourself that the way you view and ingest food is out of control, that you cannot manage your eating on a consistent basis, especially after dieting. 2) Come to the realization that an ultimate authority of spiritual magnitude will be needed to help you control your emotional eating. 3) Have belief that this ultimate authority of spiritual magnitude (the God of our choosing) could arrest your emotional eating and become willing to turn this burden over to him. Let's examine each of these three actions.

Action one is not giving up. It is admitting your way hasn't worked. Suppose you are an enterprising, industrious person, intelligent, and willing to work hard. You decide to build your own house. Remember you are hard working and intelligent; therefore, you not only will do all the sub-contracting, you are going to do some of the work yourself. You do the digging, measuring, and pouring of the foundation. Pouring and finishing the concrete proves to be trickier than you had imagined. Therefore, you do not have a level foundation. What do you do? Do you say, "Come hell or high water, I'm going to keep on going?" I don't think you would. An intelligent person would say, "I'm determined to complete this project but I am not building a crooked house. I am going to tear up this old foundation and get somebody to assist me in doing it right." That is what I am asking you to consider in part one of the surrender process. This is the deep dark secret I spoke of in Chapter One, the one you have to discover yourself. Am I ready? Am I willing to change? Do I have the courage to change? Am I sick and tired of fighting this on my own? Am I WILLING? No one can decide this but you.

Assuming you are willing, let us examine action two. This is where you are being asked to believe in something far greater than yourself and to put your trust in something that we are calling the God of your choosing. This means it does not have to be the God of the Bible. You do not have to profess any one particular religion. You don't even have to be religious; but you do have to be spiritual.

You also have to be WILLING to conclude that this power will be required to help you. Your God will have to help do for you what you have not been able to do yourself. Even if you are an agnostic, or an atheist this action will work. However, you must pray to this power whether imaginary or real and ask for help. Of course if you are a believer in God, it makes it a lot easier for you to take this action. There are many people who are believers that do not belong to any segment of organized religion nor do they attend a mass, synagogue, or church. And how about those Deists who believe more in the order of the universe by reason rather than faith or a revealed religion?

It will work for you all. The only thing required is a WILLINGNESS to be open and make the effort. There will be those of you, who like me, have struggled with emotional eating all of their lives who will say; oh, I have prayed about this before, for years, and God did not answer my prayers. My answer to you is this: God gave you intelligence that distinguishes us humans from all other creatures on earth. Do you think in my earlier example of the man that was building the house that praying about his mistake would have miraculously created a level foundation? The God of our choosing has provided us with the intelligence to say I did not do this right. I'm going to get help and start over.

Step number three in the surrender process is a real ego buster. Remember the example of the foundation? There what we needed to do was tear down before we built back up. Any exercise specialist will tell you that in order to build muscle you have to exercise it to failure. The rebuilding process does not begin while you are in the gym. It begins after you have left the gym. Then and only then with rest and proper nourishment does your muscle begin to grow.

The same happens with your mind. When you turn this emotional eating problem over to the God of your choosing, your mind is at rest and it will grow as long as you pray asking for help and guidance with your eating problem. That is additional nourishment that your brain will need as well as the healthy food that you will be feeding your body. This was covered in the chapter on Eating Healthy.

In this chapter, I have given you a lot more than food to digest. I am not asking you to do anything I have not done as illustrated in Chapter Two: My Story. I suggest you find a spiritual advisor to guide you through the three action steps of the surrender process. After the surrender process, the real fun part is about to start. It's time for some real soul searching! We are going to rid ourselves of the toxins, the poisons that keep us addicted to food. This is the psychological aspect of the problem we are addressing now. We are going to call the totality of this exercise "The Brain Flush."

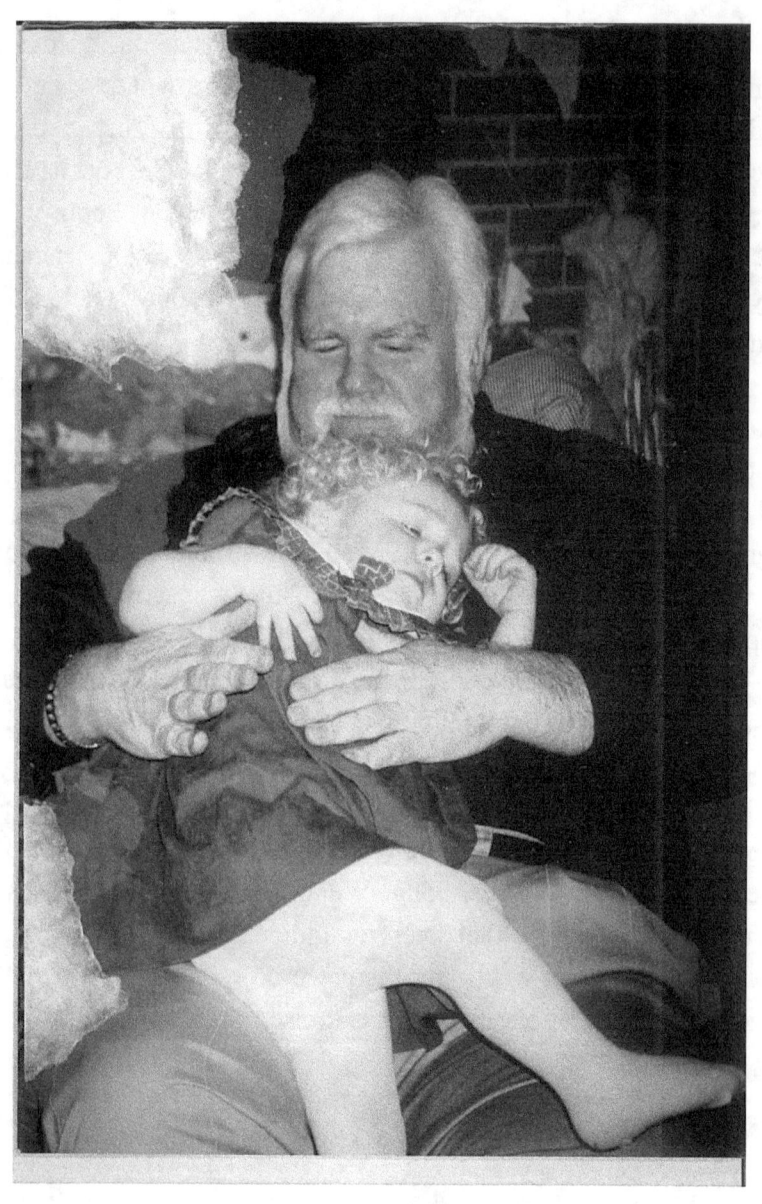

Chapter Eleven
The Brain Flush

In order to rid ourselves of resentments and fears, the brain flush exercise is absolutely essential. When we hang on to these resentments and fears, it causes pain, sometimes subconsciously. All of us have been in stressful situations that demanded a lot of us emotionally. While we are going through these, it doesn't seem to affect us that much because we are doing what we know we have to do; therefore, we subconsciously push out the concurrent pain associated with our ordeal. And when it is over, there may be some temporary relief, but eventually the avalanche comes down upon you.

An example for me was my wife's diagnosis of a brain cancer, called glioblastoma. The surgeon told me it was almost always fatal and that the patient would live about nine months. I always tried to put on a good face for her and I cherished the time we were able to spend together. During those nine months, I pushed out the pain, sometimes with food, and sometimes with alcohol. But when it was all over, I felt as if I had been hit by a freight train. The pain was at times unbearable and I needed comfort from it. Despair, self-pity, anger, resentment, and fear were my constant companions. Seven months after Judy's death, I had a heart attack and triple bypass surgery. A little less than two years after that, I discovered these principles and put them into action. The brain flush played a big part in my recovery from food addiction. What I am about to tell you is what I did.

This exercise freed me from myself, from holding on to fears and resentments that I had kept hidden for a long time. Although recalling unpleasant memories was somewhat painful, the spiritual awakening and freedom I felt after "The Brain Flush" was totally euphoric. It enabled me to move forward with my life, a life that now had newfound purpose. I was able to reconcile the past and take responsibility for the future.

The first things we need to address are resentments. We need to list them in a column, one under another. List everything you can think of that has made you angry, resentful, threatened or hurt. These are usually people: But they can be institutions, ideas, or principles. For example, some people are mad at God or the Church.

After you have completed listing all the resentments you can think of, in a second column, across from each resentment, list the cause. Specifically explain what happened and why you were angry. In another column, which would be column number three across from two, list how this made you feel. Note how it affected the seven parts of self. Following are the definitions of the seven parts of self:

1. Self-Esteem—how I think of me
2. Sex Relations—basic drive for sexual intimacy
3. Ambition—goals and plans for the future
4. Pride—how I perceive others to view me
5. Financial—basic desire for money, property, and possessions
6. Personal Relations—relationships with other people
7. Emotional Security—sense of personal well being

Here is an additional listing of some areas that have caused resentment in others: Marriage, Bible, Church, Religion, Races, Law, Authority, Government, Education System, Philosophy, and Nationality. Additionally, here are some principles that may be helpful in your inventory: God, Deity, Retribution, Ten Commandments, Jesus Christ, Satan, Death, Life after death, Heaven, Hell, Sin, Adultery, Golden Rule, or The Seven Deadly Sins.

Remember to list all your resentments in a column. Across from that resentment of a person, institution or principle, list the cause. Tell why you were/are angry, then in a column across from that how it affected the seven parts of self.

In the next column, which will be column number four, describe anything you could have done differently. Describe where you may have played a part in the outcome of the situation and why it happened this way. Search for any responsibility you may have had in this, and was there anything you could have done to change the end result. Identify anywhere you may have been at fault.

Next you need to make a new list. This is a list of your fears. There are so many fears that people have; but here are some of the most common ones: fear of dying, fear of being alone, fear of responsibility, fear of change, fear of failure, fear of success, fear of physical pain, fear of unemployment, and fear of poverty. List your fears in a column as you did your resentments and across from them list why you have that fear.

You have now taken a personal inventory of yourself, something like you have never done before. When a business owner takes an inventory, it tells that person a lot about the condition of the business. Having the right merchandise in the right amount facilitates a more efficient and profitable operation for the owner. It will be the same for you as a person. You will be able to identify your character flaws as well as maybe for the first time identify these demons that are literally keeping you from losing weight and keeping it off.

I know this is quite a task that I am asking of you for I have done it and done it meticulously. Take your time. Be thorough. Be truthful. And now it is confession time. Get ready to sing like a canary and spill the beans.

This part of the brain flush involves confession. After I completed this part of the brain flush, I really understood what the expression "confession is good for the soul" meant. A feeling of euphoric and cleansing proportions was infused into me. Do you remember the devastation and calamity of Hurricane Katrina and how it was reported on television? Almost every reporter from every network said something like this on reporting for his or her first time live from the scene. You cannot experience the real magnitude of this catastrophe from viewing it on television. By witnessing the aftermath live, you can truly feel the devastation and its impact on the survivors that experienced it. The reporters had felt this from the inside out. You could hear the emotion in all of their voices.

This is the kind of reaction you will have by sharing your list of resentments and fears with a live person. Whether you are Catholic or not, a priest is a great support structure to discuss your lists with. Any clergy trained for spiritual counseling will work, or even your best friend can hear your confession. Whomever you choose should be someone who is trusting and respectful of your privacy and confidentiality. Discussing things with another person gives you clarity that you cannot receive in any other way. The fact that you are telling someone some things about yourself that you have probably never discussed with anyone relieves you of a feeling of loneliness that you may have been harboring without willfully recognizing it.

I think all of us real overeaters know that loneliness, a feeling that we are different and don't quite belong. The biggest objection from doing this part of "the Brain Flush" sometimes comes from God-fearing, religious folks. There are certain things I want to keep between my maker and me. Besides, God is all-powerful, and in the case of a Christian, "all things are possible through Christ." My answer to this is even the most devout and learned of spiritual advisors get advice and feedback from other people. Everyone can use a sounding board.

Since this is a spiritual movement we are discussing, let me see if I can put this into better perspective by sharing my own spiritual experience. I pray to the God Of My Choosing every day asking for His guidance and will for me. I had asked My God many times before to help me with my overeating problem. I never got a clear answer until I did all of the "Brain Flush." Once I did the brain flush I could see that God had His hand in directing me to a program that taught me this confessional technique. Once I confessed and discussed these things with another person, I destroyed the list. There is no need to revisit it. This confession to another person I believe to be the catalyst for the expulsion of the obsession to overeat.

Your selection of the person to share your very personal information with, as you may imagine, must be someone who is not going to judge you. That is not their job. You are not due a dissertation on morality. This person is helping you to remove and pick up the garbage. It is necessary to forgive those who have harmed you. Carrying resentment against someone is like poisoning yourself to watch him or her die. Be as forgiving as possible, and by the way, if you have harmed someone, then that needs to be addressed as well. Apologize and make amends if possible. It is not a perfect world; therefore, you may have harmed someone that will not forgive you. As long as you have tried, that is what is important. Remember, we cannot control what others do; only what we do.

The Brain Flush is a suggested course of action that I recommend to anyone that thinks they have a food addiction. Humanity would be well served if every human being did the Brain Flush. However, as a weight loss specialist and life coach, I do not demand this of my clients. If the willingness to participate is not there, we proceed without it. Certainly weight loss can still be achieved, even permanently. Without The Brain Flush, the chance of maintaining permanent weight loss is simply reduced.

Now we know that if we choose to create a new and fresh start on our weight loss outlook, doing the Brain Flush will help us immeasurably in controlling our emotional eating.

To review chapters ten and eleven and the seven principles, first we surrender our old ways by admitting to ourselves that our eating is out of control, that we are emotional eaters. Then we come to realize that there is a power beyond our comprehension, the God of our choosing, who we need to help us manage our emotions and lives. We give ourselves willingly to our God to manage our weight problem. Next we made a list of resentments, fears, and people we need to forgive and people we may have harmed. We then discuss and share all this information with another person; and make amends to anyone we may have harmed without causing further harm.

I suggest that you review in its entirety the instructions on how to do the Brain Flush, prepare meticulously then ready, fire, aim. Here's the URL for my website where you can find the worksheets: www.stevetaylormyownweigh.com and go to the services section.

Chapter Twelve
Getting Started

Throughout this book, there are some pretty explicit instructions on becoming mentally prepared to a new and fresh approach to weight loss. There is also a suggested eating plan for the first six weeks, including cutting back portions of what you are currently eating the first two weeks, then The Three Bears Diet the next four weeks, then starting one of the diets I critiqued after that. All of these recommendations are based upon my vast experience of dieting, food knowledge, and my psychological understanding of behavioral eating. But what do you need to get started? Can you start taking action on your own? For many people this is quite difficult. In fact for most people it is quite difficult. I help people with this journey as a professional coach, counselor, and teacher.

What is coaching? Take a piece of notebook paper. Turn it sideways so the 11-inch side is horizontal rather than vertical. From left to right, draw five 1-1/2 inch rectangles. In the first one, write down your weight loss goal, in the second write how long you have had this goal, in the third write what is keeping you from this goal, in the fourth write what you have done to work toward this goal, in the fifth and last rectangle write what will be the result of your completing your goal? How will it make you feel? Now, look at the fifth and last rectangle and focus on it only. Isn't that really your goal?

After you have done this exercise, I hope you internalized a coaching experience. It is easier to have a coaching experience than a coaching education. A good coach will help you to find within you what is good and what is not so good. A coach is like a guide that enhances the experience of the explorer. By shining the light in all the right places, the coach will help you discover self-truth, reframe your perspectives, and have the right structures that create the foundation to ensure action and success.

It would probably take several books to cover and explain coaching thoroughly; however, it is how you as a client can benefit from coaching that matters. A really skilled coach can help you on your weight loss journey. It is a wonderful structure to have. Being coached is an opportunity to partner with someone who can help bring out the best in you while acknowledging your wins and achievements, and maybe most importantly instill in you accountability and discernibility.

I, as a coach, also have my own coach, Sunita, from India. She is very experienced and skilled. A very compassionate person, she coaches from the heart. Sunita has an amazing ability to ask the right questions of me at the right time in our coaching sessions. I will not get into the specifics of our private coaching session here nor will I divulge any details of her questioning; however, in general, this is what happened.

I was struggling with the completion of a project. I didn't know exactly the direction I wanted to take to complete this project and I was overwhelmed by the enormity of the information before me. I was struggling! Sunita asked me one question and a light bulb went off in my head, an aha moment. I then knew exactly how I wanted to proceed. This serves to prove at times we all need a little help from our friends. We can all use a coach.

A counselor is simply someone who listens and gives advice. While a coach is more concerned with partnering with you to a future destination, a counselor helps to analyze your current situation and offers opinions on improving that situation or an alternative to it.

A teacher or mentor is a person who educates another individual on a particular subject. As the old saying goes, if you really want to help someone, don't just give them a fish, teach them how to fish.

The commonality of a coach, counselor, and teacher is that they all help people. I call myself a weight loss specialist. As a weight loss specialist, I wear all three hats. I am a coach, a counselor, and a teacher. I am one of the truly fortunate people in life to be serving my life's purpose, to help people who are suffering from obesity as I did for so many years. If you think you may be interested in my services, you may find me at stevetaylormyownweigh.com. For more frequent updates and information, my blog can be found on that website as well.

I wish to thank each of you who purchased *My OWN Weigh* and offer you sincerest wishes for a successful and permanent weight loss.

Thanks for listening!
Steve Taylor
My OWN Weigh

For more information and to sign up for my blog, visit me at stevetaylormyownweigh.com.

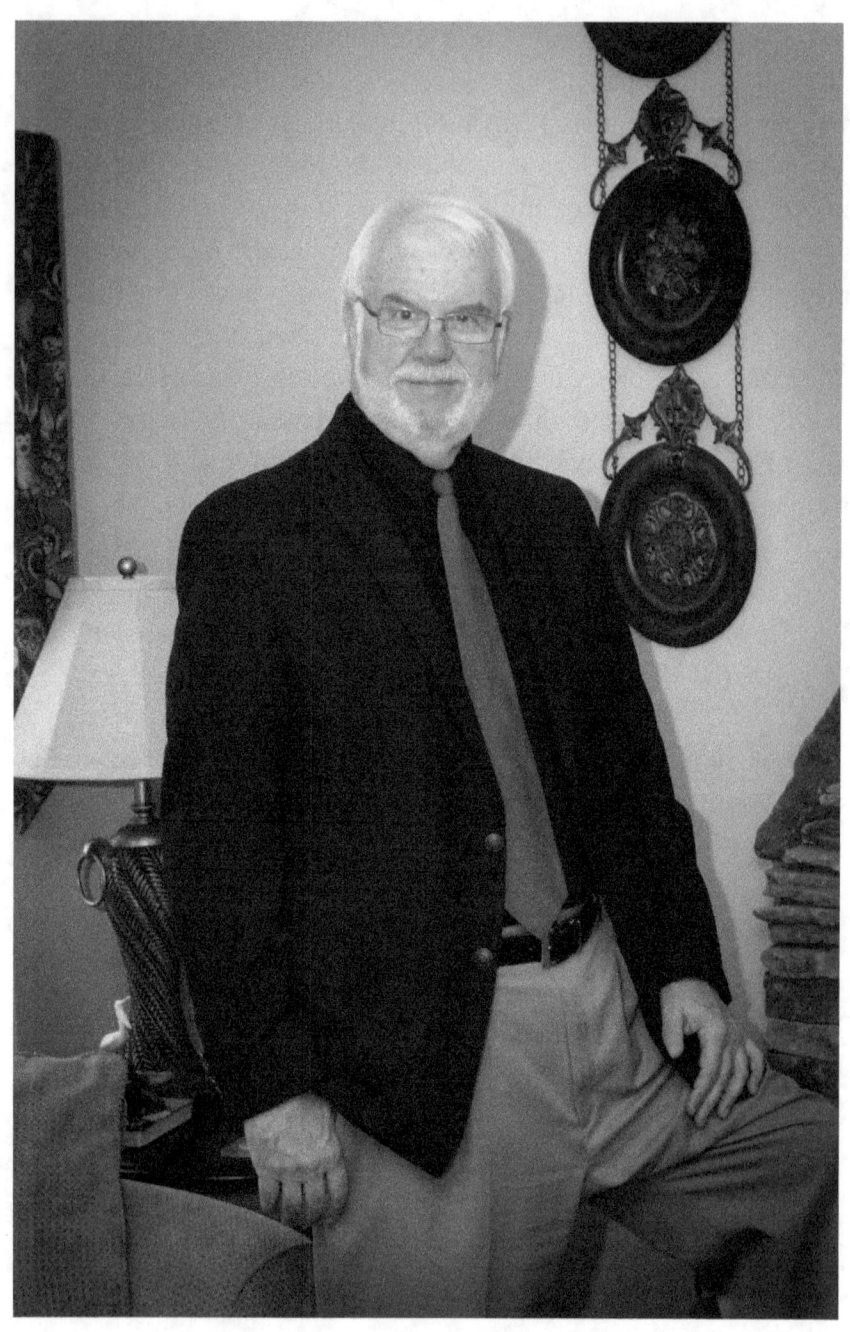

Addendum 1

Coaching Case Study

The following is a case study including conversations between my friend and client, Jenny, and me. Take a few minutes and read, and see if you can identify with Jenny's experience. You'll also get some insight into my coaching style, and what it's like to work with me to gain control over the emotional eating in your life. (Of course, names have been changed to protect the privacy of my clients.)

{Two friends are talking}...

Gerry:

Can you believe it? There we are, Gerome and Jennifer, on our wedding day. The wedding dress was about a six or eight. Today she wears a 22, but really needs a 24. Jenny is so big that if we meet in the hallway at home, it is easier to go over her than go around her.

Joe:

Gerry, do you stay on her case about losing this weight? If you do, you're probably making things worse, you know?

Gerry:

I know. Believe me I try not to, but it drives me crazy. I can keep my mouth shut for a while, but then I erupt, sometimes with volcanic intensity. I want to help her. I love her! She has been on every diet out there. We could open a bookstore on diet books alone. It is always the same song, second verse. All the diets seem to work for her, but she always gains the weight back she lost, and even a little more.

Joe:

Has she had counseling or weight loss coaching?

Gerry:

I'm not sure what that is, but she worked with a nutritionist for several weeks and a personal trainer at the gym. It worked for a while. That was a couple of years ago. I don't know exactly how much she spent, but I strongly suspect it was over $2,000. Now she has gotten so big she won't even go into a gym. She doesn't know I know, but she weighs 265. She is twice the size of the 5' 6" beauty in that wedding picture.

Joe:

Gerry, I'm no psychologist or psychiatrist, but it sure makes sense that it is a psychological problem. I am currently seeing a girl who has lost 120 pounds by working with a weight loss coach. The coach has written a book about his life long struggle with emotional eating and food addiction. According to my girlfriend, he says that maybe it is not what you are eating but what is eating you.

Gerry:

Is he some kind of counselor?

Joe:

Yes, but he is more than that. My girlfriend Cindy swears by him. Like Jenny, Cindy could never keep her weight off after dieting. She was extremely frustrated until she found this man. She says he saved her life. Would you like me to find out more about him?

Gerry:

Absolutely! I am willing to try anything to help her, and I think she will be willing also. Here is my card. When you find out more, give me a call on that cell phone. Between 3 p.m. and 5 p.m. is a good time to catch me.

THREE WEEKS LATER ...

Jenny:

Hello, Mr. Taylor?

Steve T:

Yes, this is Steve.

Jenny:

Well, hi Steve. This is Jenny, the friend of Cindy who set this consultation call up for me.

Steve T:

Yes, Jenny, I was expecting your call and I welcome it. How are you?

Jenny:

Fine, I guess. {short pause} Actually, as Cindy may have told you, I am really not fine. I am miserable. My eating is out of control; therefore, my weight is probably now twice what it should be. I have no self-esteem. My cholesterol is too high, the bad cholesterol that is, and the good cholesterol is too low. I know that means I don't exercise enough, but how can I? It hurts too much to exercise. Besides, even though I try to sit down to work on patients, I am on my feet a lot. I am afraid this weight may be affecting my patient care. I have to do something about it!

I'm a dentist by the way, in case Cindy didn't tell you and people hate dentists anyway. Did you know that? I know, I know, I am just rambling. But other than all that and feeling completely worthless, I am just fine...I guess!

{Fifteen seconds of silence}...

Steve T:

Jenny, in spite of all that, you have an acknowledgement coming, in fact you have several. First through this self-described misery of yours, you have retained something very important, your sense of humor. What a great weapon to have in your arsenal.

Secondly, you are a dentist. I say this because this is a profession that serves a very necessary niche in human health. You know, Jenny, there are about seven billion people on planet Earth. What percentage of those persons could qualify to become a dentist? You are in an elite group of persons that possess the necessary intelligence, determination, and willingness to help people that a dentist must have. Having known a few dentists pretty well over my lifetime, my Uncle was one, I know that a lot of people do dread going to the dentist, but do they really hate them? However, it is not uncommon for you to feel that way. It comes with the profession.

And Jenny, the last thing that I want to commend you and acknowledge you for is that you realize that you need help. This is what we call getting out of denial. And since I have spoken about what is uncommon and what is not uncommon, let me briefly speak further to that. What is common is for people to stay in denial about their weight and their inability to maintain weight loss after dieting. You, Jenny, sound like you realize that you could use some help. Am I interpreting that correctly?

Jenny:

Yes, you are. My friend Cindy speaks highly of you. She says you really helped her in ways that nobody else ever has. That is why I am calling you. I don't think I can handle another failure with another diet. I haven't read your book yet, but I suppose that from what I have heard, you are second to none when it comes to struggles with weight loss.

Frankly Steve, I feel desperate. I am willing and open to trying something different. But I did want to talk to you, get to know you a little, and find out a little more about how you would work with me. Cindy praised you, but she described your methods in generic terms. She said it would be best if the specifics of working with you would be discussed between the two of us.

Steve T:

Absolutely. I want to tell you how I work and explain the model for my coaching. Also in this consultation I want to cover the specifics of our contractual relationship including what you can expect from me and what I expect from you, and then, if you feel comfortable with everything, we will begin your flight to go out and bite the stars, and I mean that almost literally. That may not sound so extravagant when you discover the new you!

Now before we get into the coaching model and specifics, allow me to once again allude to something I said earlier. It is without a doubt the most important thing for you to remember from our conversation today. Jenny, you have mustered the courage to change by being WILLING and OPEN to participate in a new approach to weight loss. You are 60% there, sounds incredible, but true. If you remain willing and open and follow the suggested program, you will have about a 95% chance to complete the remaining 40% and stop the emotional eating roller coaster. Do you believe me?

Jenny:

Well...I guess I do. You certainly sound confident. I am just not so confident right now.

{Laughter from Steve}...

Steve T:

Jenny, I just used that for shock value! I don't expect you to have total confidence in yourself right now, or complete trust in me for that matter. However, I sense in you a desire to succeed, and I truly believe you will.

Now here is a little bit about how I work. First, know that I do possess a certain set of skills that can help you attain your goals by clearing up the past, and reframing your perspectives for your future. The idea is to help empower you to a life changing transformation.

I am a counselor, a mentor, and a coach. My coaching model is called SHARE. It's an acronym. The S stands for me sharing my story with you. I had wandered very deep into the woods, and there I was without a compass. I want to share with you how I got out, and if I did it at age 61, I know you can too.

The H is for your Health. The A is that we will analyze your physical and mental health and address how to deal with it. The R is where you will reframe perspectives and develop what I call a new "fooditude", (my word for food attitude). The E is that we will evaluate and execute your plan. There you have it. Describe how this sounds to you.

Jenny:

Well Steve, I don't quite understand all of it. But, it sounds very exciting, and from what Cindy says, you definitely know what you are doing.

Steve T:

I'm glad you think it is exciting, because it is very exciting. I know what I am doing because not only have I been through this myself, but for years I have helped others using this model. We will be working with a scientifically proven set of principles that have been used for more than seventy years. Jenny, in this initial consultation session there are several things that I need to explain. Do you mind if I go into those now, or do you have any questions before I get started?

Jenny:

No, please continue.

Steve T:

Okay, good. Before our first session, there is a state of health form I would like for you to fill out. I need to know when, where, what, why, and how much you are eating? The why may simply be because it is mealtime and you are hungry. I also need the other information that is related to your medical history. I'm sure as a dentist you understand my need for this information.

Additionally, there is a contractual agreement form that explains the nature of our agreement, what you can expect from me, and what I expect from you. The form is straightforward and simple and is really designed to prevent any disappointments. You can download these forms from my website, read, sign and mail them to me. My address is on the website as well. Have you looked at the website and do you have that address?

Jenny:

Yes, your website is impressive, and I have seen those forms. I will do that right away. I do have a question though. You worked with Cindy by phone. Since we are miles apart, I am assuming we will be doing the same.

Steve T:

Yes, we will. In many cases working with a client over the phone can be more effective than face to face. It really depends upon the client. Some people feel like they can be more open and forthright over the phone. How about you Jenny, are you comfortable with the phone communication?

Jenny:

Yes, I am. And Steve, I really think I am going to be comfortable with you.

Steve T:

I'm thrilled to hear that. I hope I eventually will be viewed as your new best friend. I know that is a mouthful, and it is asking for your trust. I don't expect this to happen overnight. As in any trusting relationship, it takes time to develop. For the next several weeks or months Jenny, I am going to be your guide. I hope I can shine the light in all the right places. The more open and honest you are with me, the easier it will be for me to do my job.

Jenny:

I am ready to get started. I suppose I need to send you some money.

{Slight chuckle from Steve}

Steve T:

I read the other day that money was mentioned 1500 plus times in the Bible. I suppose it has always been pretty important. I would recommend that you do the twelve-week program. For that you receive 12 one-hour coaching sessions, and six twenty-minute coaching sessions. That equates to an hour session every week and a twenty-minute session every two weeks. I usually ask for half of the fee up front to cover the first six weeks, and the other half at the beginning of the second six weeks. There are other options that cost a little more, but are you comfortable with what I recommended?

Jenny:

Yes, I am. Our dental office operates Monday through Thursday ten hours a day to make a forty-hour week. Therefore I am off on Friday. Do you have any time on Friday?

Steve T:

I have 9 a.m., 11 a.m., or 2 p.m. available on Friday. That is CST.

Jenny:

Let's do 9 a.m.

Steve T:

Okay, would you like to start this next Friday, October 5th?

Jenny:

Yes, should I call you?

Steve T:

Yes, my number is on the website.

Jenny, helping people like you fills me with joy. Let me quickly just say a couple more things. After all, this first consultation is when I talk the most. That is because although you can certainly learn something from me, in order to help you, I have to learn a lot from you. I do that by listening, not talking.

Also, this is on the contractual agreement under expectations from me, but I would like for you to hear me say it. I value the money you're paying me, the time you're giving me, and the time I'm giving you very highly. Therefore, while you're my client, I think of you often and how I can help you. Sometimes you'll receive emails from me on subjects I think may interest you or help you. I like to think of my coaching practice as a boutique. I work with a limited number of clients. I never want you to feel like I have felt before at some doctors' offices, that I was part of a cattle call.

Please download and fill out the health form and contractual agreement, mail them, and we will talk Friday.

Jenny:

I'll call you at 9 a.m. CST Friday morning.

Steve T:

Good. Goodbye Jenny. Have a good week.

Jenny:

Goodbye Steve.

SESSION ONE – FRIDAY MORNING

Steve T:

Good morning Jenny!

Jenny:

Good morning Steve. How are you?

Steve T:

Great thanks. I feel rested, and full of enthusiasm for our call. I reviewed your state of health form yesterday. Thanks for your quick response in sending it. Can you tell me some things you learned from filling it out?

Jenny:

Well, sure. I think the biggest thing I learned was just confirming the fact that I am an emotional eater. Whenever I am stressed, I eat. Whenever I am bored, I eat. And whenever there is food within my sight or reach, I am tempted. Whenever temptation comes I give right in, most of the time. And, you see what I eat. I buy those Lance peanut butter crackers by the boxes. Reese's Peanut Butter Cups would not be recommended to my patients for consumption, but I wolf them right down. As you can see, I get no exercise other than standing on my feet all day at work. Of course I do sit in a chair when I work on patients, but I am still on my feet a lot. When I get home I am tired. I don't cook much; therefore Gerome and I eat out often.

Steve T:

What I am hearing is that there are several things that are driving you to be an emotional eater, triggers that incite you to eat. When you do eat, you are eating processed sugar and fat, by your own admission not good for you, and that you don't get any proper exercise. Is that right?

Jenny:

Yes, I guess that's right. I know what I am doing is wrong but I can't do anything about it.

Steve T:

Why?

Jenny:

Why can't I do anything about it?

Steve T:

Yes.

Jenny:

Well, I... uh.... I'm not exactly sure. I guess I have never thought about it.

Steve T:

Actually, you have already done something about it. You have engaged me to help you and as I told you in our consultation session, you have recognized that you have a problem. Now do you mind if I get into a mentoring mode and share with you my thoughts on what you have told me?

Jenny:

No. Please do. I'm really at a loss to understand or explain my behavior.

Steve T:

In my view you are addicted to food, and you use food as a comfort cushion to push out emotional pain. Pain is pain, and emotional pain is real. So when you are bored, you eat. When you are stressed, you eat. The whole process of eating can be sensual and alluring. The smell and taste of food, the chewing and swallowing of food are pleasant experiences, and they block out any stress or anxiety you may be experiencing. When turning to food for comfort becomes an automatic reaction, we call this an addiction. For example, I used to find myself in the kitchen standing with the refrigerator door open without really remembering what prompted me to get up and do that. In other words, I don't remember a little voice saying, there is some leftover chicken Steve, why don't you just get up and get some? Does any of this sound familiar or make sense to you?

Jenny:

Oh yes! Before I know it, there is a Reese's Peanut Butter Cup going into my mouth, or my beloved Subway cookies, chocolate chip of course. So are you suggesting that my eating is a psychological problem?

Steve T:

I am suggesting that is part of the problem. The other part of the problem is physical. I think you have an allergy to certain foods, namely the processed foods you mentioned earlier like the crackers and candy and cookies. The more you eat them the higher your sugar levels become, requiring your pancreas to overwork to produce more insulin. As you know this can lead to Diabetes. Jenny, here is the good news! Both the psychological and physical problems you are experiencing are treatable. Remember the SHARE coaching model we talked about in your consultation a few days ago?

Jenny:

Yeah, the S stood for share as you sharing your story.

Steve T:

Exactly. In the part of my book, *My OWN Weigh*, called Steve's Story, I talk about my 1000-pound journey. Before I share some of that experience with you, I would like to just reiterate that anything you tell me is in the strictest of confidence. This refers in particular to some of the personal information you may later reveal to me. I may also reveal some personal information to you that is not in my book. I would trust that you keep that information about me in confidence. I would share this information only if it may be a mutual experience we shared, or if it was something I thought would help you. Are you still okay with this agreement of mutual trust?

Jenny:

Steve, I am okay with it. I know you covered it in your contractual agreement. Anything you wish to tell me about you that you think would help me, I will treat the same way I would treat my patient's dental records. They are not discussed with anyone but the patient, unless authorized by the patient.

Steve T:

Thank you Jenny. My story is probably best expressed by the illustration in the 1000-pound journey which is in my book and on my website. Have you seen that?

Jenny:

Yes, I have purchased the printed version of *My OWN Weigh* and have reviewed your website.

Steve T:

Good! I think reading my book will really help you. The 1000-pound journey is expressed in the narrative in the book to further enhance the illustration. That journey really speaks to what I experienced. Jenny, I really did not know what to do except try another diet. I kept looking for the panacea, the diet that would lead to nirvana. There had to be one I thought. I just had not found it yet. Finally, I came to my senses. You can see at the epiphany point on the graph what happened. Something clicked. Now, it is time to get back to you and analyze the physical part of this program. Are you ready for that?

Jenny:

Yes.

Steve T:

All right, start analyzing.

Jenny:

What? I thought you were the coach!

Steve T:

Yep. But I want to hear more of your thoughts on what you learned analyzing your eating habits. After all, you are a smart lady Jenny, smart enough to become a dentist.

Jenny:

Okay, I suppose you have your reasons for doing this, making me analyze my eating habits.

Steve T:

You would be correct. Now we are aware of the peanut butter crackers and Reese's Peanut Butter Cups. Tell me more.

Jenny:

Well, I know I eat late at night. We don't have dinner until around 9 p.m. I read a lot to relax after dinner and sometimes I even have a midnight snack, usually yogurt. I start seeing patients at 8 a.m. so I don't get up in time to eat breakfast. I usually start snacking between patients sometime around mid morning. My sweet husband prepares my sack lunch for me every day and it is usually healthy, consisting of a sandwich with only a little light mayo and a meat with lettuce tomato, some carrot or celery sticks, a dill pickle, and a piece of fruit like a banana, peach, or apple. So I suppose I should get up earlier, eat breakfast, not snack, and eat dinner earlier, right? Come on Steve, your turn to tell me something.

Steve T:

First, I have a couple of questions. What kind of meat do you eat on your sandwich, and what is the brand of yogurt you eat for a late night snack?

Jenny:

The meat is 98% fat free and comes in a package. I usually alternate between turkey, chicken, and ham. I think it is only about 45 calories per slice, or something like that. The yogurt is low fat. I think it has 180 calories, but I'm not sure.

Steve T:

How many grams of sugar are in the yogurt?

Jenny:

I don't know.

Steve T:

Check it. It could be as high as 18 grams. I prefer you not eat anything higher than 7 grams per serving. We have got to get your sugar level down and break your sugar addiction. This could be a starting point. Buy 0% fat Greek Oikos yogurt. I think it may have 8 grams of sugar per serving, but that is okay. One cup is 120 calories. I eat this myself as a snack. I sweeten it with Stevia, or the Walmart version Truvia. Squeeze part of a fresh lemon on it, and add fruit like strawberries, bananas, or apples, about a half a cup of that. You may also use low fat cottage cheese instead of the yogurt with the same formula. You may want to try it with or without the lemon. Is this something you can do?

Jenny:

Yes, I believe I will like the taste, and I do like cottage cheese as well.

Steve T:

Good. One other change I'd like you to make, stop using the processed meat. You can buy Sara Lee oven-roasted turkey at Walmart here in Alabama for $6.48 per pound. Have them slice it for you in 3-ounce servings. It is fresher, less processed than what you are eating, and actually more economical, plus it tastes a lot better. Of course, I don't know where you shop or how much it would cost in Florida, but whatever you buy, buy it freshly sliced. It will be healthier for you along with the other advantages I mentioned. Those are the first two changes I am asking for this week. Are you up for that?

Jenny:

Yes, that should not be a problem.

Steve T:

Are you up for two or three more?

Jenny:

Like what?

Steve T:

What about referring to your previous analysis?

Jenny:

You mean how late I eat dinner or skipping breakfast?

Steve T:

I mean how late you eat dinner. Changing your routine by getting up earlier and eating breakfast would not be advisable right now. I want these changes to be baby steps. You will be sprinting on down the road. Is there a good reason you can't move your dinnertime up an hour till eight?

Jenny:

I could do that.

Steve T:

Okay, that is change number three. What if I told you Jenny, that instead of one snack at midnight, you could have two, one at 10am, and one mid afternoon when you can work it in?

Jenny:

Can I still have my peanut butter cups, crackers, and cookies?

Steve T:

That would be an emphatic no! But in the spirit of true negotiation and compromise, if you give them up, you can have another sandwich, as long as it is eaten between 10 a.m. and 6 p.m.

Jenny:

Can I put a couple of slices of avocados on the sandwich? I hear they are a healthy fat.

Steve T:

Absolutely, as long as they are small to medium slices, but no mayo, just mustard. Are you okay with that?

Jenny:

Steve, did you know that mayo makes things taste better?

Steve T:

Jenny did you know that you can put a small amount of extra virgin olive oil on your bread, and then you have that taste you are referring to, but with a healthy fat? Just a few drops is all it takes. You can either dip your knife in it and spread it on the slices of bread, or mix it with vinegar and put it on your lettuce and tomato.

Jenny:

Okay, Steve, I will do that. Let me just make sure I got what we have discussed written down correctly. I am changing the brand of yogurt I am eating to reduce the sugar content. I am also changing the time I eat it, no more midnight snacks. I can also have cottage cheese, low fat cottage cheese with about a half a cup of fruit, and I can put the fruit in with the yogurt as well. I can have two of those snacks per day.

Now when it comes to my sandwich or what is now my sandwich and a half, I drop the processed meat, buy fresh turkey sliced at the deli, and make my sandwich without mayo, but may add a little avocado, mustard, olive oil, or veggies if I wish. I have to eat this sandwich and a half between 10 a.m. and 6 p.m. every day. Do I have that right so far?

Steve T:

It sounds good except for one little thing about the veggies. I wish you would make those mandatory for your sandwich. Maybe I heard you wrong, but you seem to imply those were optional. I thought you said add them if you wish. The veggies contain fiber and a whole lot of nutrients that you need. I am sorry I did not make that clearer earlier.

Jenny:

Okay, gotcha! Oh, and the last thing we talked about was moving my dinner earlier to 8 p.m.

Steve T:

Jenny, you are now right on target. Now, just a couple more minor changes for this week. One, watch your portion sizes at dinner, reduce them about fifteen per cent of what they are now. Two, increase your intake of water, not to the point you are uncomfortable, just increase it. Are you on board with those changes?

Jenny:

I am. I think I can implement the changes we discussed without sacrifice. Do you think I will lose weight the first week by making those changes?

Steve T:

My experience tells me that you will, but let's find out. Since tomorrow is not a workday, I would like for you to weigh yourself stripped first thing in the morning after voiding. That is how you will weigh every week to maintain the accuracy of your weight loss. Also measuring is important. It is good to have someone like your husband to assist you. Measure your neck, chest, waist, and hips. Also measure your upper arms with them hanging at your sides, your thighs, calves, and ankles. Then, you get to choose your own wardrobe for your picture taking. Any thoughts on what you might wear?

Jenny:

{Jenny gets the subtle humor on the wardrobe question and chuckles;}

Steve, all I know is it will not be designer jeans, form fitting, or a two-piece bathing suit. Jenny laughs again.

Steve T:

I love that sense of humor of yours Jenny. Whatever you want to wear is fine, just be sure you get the picture taken now. My heaviest before picture is about 425 pounds, while my all time high was 440 pounds. When people ask me do you have any pictures of yourself at 440 pounds, I usually answer this way. Do you see a lot of big fat people lined up at Olan Mills to get their picture made? I am glad that others found the occasion to take pictures of me at Christmas, etc. when I was extremely heavy. I think it helps me now to look at them every once in a while. Sometimes, it is hard to imagine that I was that person. Looking at those pictures keeps me entrenched in the principles that afforded me my transformation. It also makes me feel humbled and grateful for what has happened. Jenny, I want you to experience the same thing I have experienced.

Jenny:

Steve, I will have several pictures taken in several different outfits, put them on a disc, and forward them to you for safekeeping. Now back to my diet. Wouldn't it be a good idea if I wrote down my meal plan for the week and send that to you along with the pictures?

Steve T:

Jenny, I have to acknowledge you for the initiative you are showing as a client. Your attitude is superb. Keep it up and before long, the new Jenny will emerge.

THE REST OF THE SESSION

Much of the rest of the first coaching session was spent discussing Jenny's new diet with me answering questions, but asking Jenny if she could hold back on the throttle until we make sure the engine is running properly. Jenny is highly intelligent, an achiever, and by nature a curious person.

Being also a driven person, Jenny is a little impatient with the pace of her diet restructuring. Although as a coach, my desire is that Jenny dictates how the sessions go, or as we say in coaching, meeting her in her journey, I know that you can come out of the starting blocks too fast. This is best illustrated by the example of Leon and the mile run in the chapter in my book on "How To Start On A Diet." Therefore, I want to keep Jenny grounded and focused on small changes in her diet that will have a big impact on her recovery.

SESSION TWO – WEEK TWO

Most of Session Two involved Jenny discussing the impact of the small changes she made in her diet. She was ecstatic that she had lost FIVE pounds the first week. She made all of the changes that were discussed in Session One without experiencing any hunger or deprivation. The sugar and fat she had been eating contained in the candy and crackers was beginning to flush out of her body. I cautioned Jenny about setting expectations for that kind of a weight loss every week. Even though I knew that Jenny was aware after so many diet attempts that her weight loss would slow down, I want to keep her more focused on improving her health and serving her body nutritionally. If Jenny can concentrate on developing an exemplary attitude about food, then her fooditude (food attitude) will change resulting in an automatic weight loss.

Some changes were made in the evening meal. The first week the portion size was reduced by 15%. In week two Jenny was introduced to the Three Bears Diet. Jenny had read *My OWN Weigh* and was familiar with the diet. She is now going to portion her food with the palm of her hand. She will also minimize the frequency of eating starchy carbs during the week, as she would usually have corn, potatoes, and rice every night. These veggies have been limited to three times per week. The primary vegetables eaten at night are broccoli, spinach, turnip greens, kale, and other green leafy vegetables. These are vegetables that Jenny enjoys and that she has selected to eat. It was Jenny's idea to go on The Three Bears Diet. What I am doing in Session Two is customizing that diet exclusively for Jenny, including the three weekly cheat snacks or one weekly meal off the program.

It is important to note that each client has a customized eating program. That is the crux of *My OWN Weigh*. Each person must own his or her diet. Jenny owns her program. Here are other changes that were made.

Daily, Jenny will drink six glasses of water (excluding other beverages containing water such as coffee or tea). She will have three servings of whole grains daily, three servings of vegetables, three servings of lean protein, two servings of fruit, two healthy fats, two dairy, and two snacks. And, by the way, Jenny has chosen for her free meal this week New York Strip and baked potato with vegetable medley. She has agreed to lightly dress her potato with butter, salt, and pepper. She is having death by chocolate for dessert but has promised to split it with her husband. The Strip will not be the largest one. Jenny has agreed to abide by my philosophy of pigleting out, not pigging out.

SESSION THREE – THE START OF THE BRAIN FLUSH

{Jenny and Steve are on the phone}

Jenny inquires:

Steve, haven't I essentially done the first three steps? I have admitted my eating is unmanageable, and that I need an authority of ultimate magnitude to help me. I have also agreed to turn my life over to this ultimate authority that I am calling God. So I guess I am asking is there anything to be discussed here or can we just get right in to talking about my resentments and fears. I have made a list of them on the forms you provided on your website. I never knew I had so many resentments and fears.

Steve T:

Jenny, I would like to discuss the first three steps with you. That would provide some validation for me to where you are in the program. I feel very comfortable with you from what I have learned through our conversations about steps one and two, but would you mind in your own words describing how you view these first two steps?

Jenny:

Sure, I know from my painful experiences of always regaining my lost weight that my eating is unmanageable. For years my ego and intellect have been battling. For years my ego has been winning, and for no good reason, other than letting my pride and false self-esteem play mind tricks on me. But when I get out of myself and stand back to take a look, my intellect says, Jenny, you are not seeing the forest for the trees. After years of trying all different kinds of diets, my intellect has put the brakes on me. The futility of not being able to maintain a weight loss has drained me emotionally. I have bottomed out Steve and I know I need some kind of divine interference to help me.

Steve T:

Thank you for sharing that Jenny. That was well said. You mentioned earlier that you have turned your life over to God. I would like to ask Jenny, not for the purpose of judging you, but for the purpose of understanding your spiritual foundation, who is your God? Is it the God of the Bible that is omnipotent and omniscient?

Jenny:

Yes, I believe in the God of the Bible. I am a Christian by faith. My husband and I are Methodists. We attend Church regularly, tithe, and we sing in the choir.

Steve T:

You clarified that for me. For your information, the reason I am asking is that our spiritual condition plays a very important role in our recovery from food addiction. May I share a little of my experience with you.

Jenny:

Please do.

Steve T:

Know the condition I was in. I prayed to God for guidance, and through a strange set of circumstances including a new person coming out of nowhere into my life, I was encouraged to get into this program.

I applied myself to following the principles we are working now and prayed for guidance and God's will for me as I worked these steps. It is important for me to mention this to you to emphasize that this is a spiritual program. It is not a religious program in the sense that it matters what faith you follow or what institution houses and hosts your faith. This program has created a new purpose in life for me and has brought me serenity and peace. Those are qualities I had sought but never could find before.

Jenny:

WOW! Everybody I know is looking for serenity and peace. I guess when I find it I will have addressed emotional eating. And you know Steve, I am beginning to feel something I have never felt before. I can't really describe it yet, but I think I am growing spiritually.

Steve T:

I can feel the vibes Jenny. Let us see if we can go a little deeper. You have indicated that you have done your resentment and fears list. Shall we get started?

Jenny:

Well...I have started. It's a little painful Steve. I guess I am putting it off. Do you have any suggestions?

Steve T:

I have a tooth that needs filling. I cancelled my last appointment. I guess I am afraid it could be a little painful, any suggestions?

Jenny:

Steve, don't cleverly manipulate me with logic. This is "emotional eating" you know.

Steve T:

Okay, let's do some right and left brainwork, Jenny. Take a minute here, and I do mean a minute and meditate. Envision the future you from head to toe, how you will look when you see your reflection in the mirror. Will you do this?

Jenny:

Okay, I will.

{One minute later}

Jenny:

Steve, I looked awfully good. I finally visualized the transformation.

Steve T:

Great! You have just practiced some creative visualization. We will do more of that later.

Jenny is the decision to postpone your step work going to get you there or is there a better way?

Jenny:

Thanks, you have made your point. You are disappointed in me aren't you? I did lose another three pounds this week you know.

Steve T:

I am proud of your weight loss, eight pounds in two weeks. Jenny, there is more in you than the procrastination you are showing today. You have the heart of a lion. I am very impressed with you in every respect. I suppose I always expect the very best from you. Maybe my expectations of you are too high. What do you think?

Jenny:

Steve, you are right to expect the very best in me. I have prepared my resentments and fears list like I said I would. I won't disappoint you. I will do this. We can start by discussing my biggest resentment.

Steve T:

I cherish the fact that I hold some accountability for you. However, Jenny, I am really not surprised that you are reluctant to share your list. The first time I prepared my list was not the last. I revised it because I simply did not want to reveal some things about myself to my confidant. Your apprehension is natural and certainly has been felt by many others before you who have gone through this process. Now, let me hear about your major resentment.

Jenny:

It's actually two family members, my brother and my father. My brother is two years my senior and he was the apple of my father's eye so to speak. Both of them are highly intelligent and are gifted in math, physics, and science. I am not. Both of them have won prestigious honors in their field, I have not. I always felt inferior to them and unworthy when comparing my accomplishments to theirs.

My father was disappointed to hear that I was going to go to dental school. At one time I expressed my desire to him to be some kind of surgeon, and would choose my specialty later. He thought I had copped out when I chose to become a lowly Dentist. He had very high expectations of me. He is a very stoic man. I did see him cry once when my Mother died. Other than that, it is certainly safe to say that he is not emotional. He views my emotional eating problem as a sign of weakness.

I think, Steve that he views himself as the strong overachiever, and his daughter as the weak underachiever.

Steve T:

Tell me about your Mother Jenny, and when did she die?

Jenny:

Mother was amazing! She would have to be to please my Father. I think he adored her. He respected her. She was a marvelous cook, a classical pianist, and vocalist. She was an instructor in piano and voice. She was an excellent teacher. Mother was a contestant on Jeopardy. She was the champion for one show, but then got dethroned. My Father was awfully proud of her. I think he loved her deeply.

Steve T:

How did they meet?

Jenny:

{Laughter.}

It was like a classical movie scene. Mother was playing with a small ensemble at a wedding reception. During the break, she went to get a bit of the bubbly. My Father was in front of her at the bar. When he turned around awkwardly holding four champagne glasses, the spill occurred, right down the front of Mother's dress. And, right into the cleavage formed by Mother's endowment. She was a full D. According to Mom, my Father was speechless, aghast, and staring at Mother's breast. Mother had the presence of mind to say. "You seem perplexed. Don't worry. I think there is more champagne, or are you simply enjoying the view?"

See, I told you it was classic!

Steve T:

Jenny, that is classic! It does sound like something written for a movie script. Later, I would like to hear more about their story. It is fascinating. But for now, I would like to get back to your resentment. What I hear you saying is that your resentment of your Father partly is based on his lack of affection shown toward you and his failure to recognize and acknowledge your accomplishments. Additionally, it appears this may have created a fear in you that you would never be able to meet his expectations. Therefore, you would always fall short of pleasing him. Is that right?

Jenny:

That is exactly right. This resentment has also created a fear.

Steve T:

Yes, resentments always create fears. Think about this Jenny. Anger, resentment, and fear are really closely related to being the same emotion. Anger is the present tense, resentment is the past tense that we tend to rewind and replay over and over, so that the future tense fear is created.

Jenny, this seems to be your major resentment and fear. Getting rid of this would help your emotional eating. Is there any reason you would like to hang on to this resentment, or are you ready to get rid of it?

Jenny:

I have hung on to it long enough. How do I, or you, make it go away?

Steve T:

Only you can make it go away. I will provide you with a technique to do that...but first a couple of questions. Can you think of something special your Father has done for you? The second question is do you think in any way you could have had a small part in the current status of your relationship?

Jenny:

Well, I'll answer your last question first because I know that is on my resentment form, and I have been thinking about it. When Mother died a couple of years ago, Gerome and I did not stay with my Father, we stayed in a motel nearby. Although he acted like that was okay, I think it hurt his feelings. My Brother and his wife were staying there, and he and my Father are so close…I just did not want to stay there. I see now where that was a mistake.

My Father and Brother did do something special for me. They deeded their share of the family condo over to me. It is a very nice beach property in Destin, Florida. Mother was very frugal with her money and over the years had saved enough to purchase it as an investment. It is an easy drive for us and we use it often as well as rent it and share it with friends.

Steve T:

Thanks for sharing Jenny. Now here is what I would like for you to do. Since you are regularly praying, I would like for you to pray intently for your Father. I would like for you to get on your knees and pray for all the good wishes for your Father that you would wish for yourself, such as health, wealth, and happiness. I also suggest that you pray for his forgiveness for anything that you may have done to offend him, and pray for your acceptance of him as he is, and for your resentment of him to be removed. Do this every day intently for thirty days! Will you do that?

Jenny:

I will start today.

REMAINDER OF SESSION THREE AND SESSIONS FOUR, FIVE, AND SIX

These sessions were spent discussing in detail all of Jenny's resentments and fears. Jenny unloaded all of her baggage. There is no longer any need to sweep these things under the rug. She has forgiven herself and others and has become willing to ask for forgiveness from her forgiveness list and make amends when possible.

Jenny has commented to me that she has never had such a euphoric spiritual feeling that she now possesses. Her acceptance of life on its terms is based upon God's will for her. She feels that no matter what happens things will work out for her. The really neat thing is that when there is so little emotional pain, there is no need to deal with it through food.

SESSION SEVEN

Steve T:

Jenny, with your permission, can we start talking about reframing your perspectives, your support structures, and maybe even try some visualization?

Jenny:

Yeah, what's first?

Steve T:

You tell me.

Jenny:

Let's do some visualization. You know I am doing some meditating on my own.

Steve T:

I know. Let's try something. If you are not already, sit somewhere comfortable in a supportive position. Picture yourself somewhere alone surrounded by mountains on the oceanfront. Breathe from your diaphragm like a newly born baby would, like your Mother would teach in her vocal class. Take slow deliberate breaths concentrating on nothing but your breathing and the sound of the ocean waves. Make sure you are bare-footed, let your feet touch the water. Close your eyes. Feel your feet and lower body becoming one with nature. Allow a tingling, relaxing feeling to creep up your legs. Feel it slowly flow from your toes all the way to the top of your head. Take a minute to thoroughly experience this...

With positive energy and your eyes closed let your imagination flow. See yourself climbing the mountain with ease and without fear. All you are hearing are birds chirping, waves roaring, and the wind whispering. You are completely at peace. Your destination is the top of the mountain where you will find a village, the village of your dreams. What will it look like? What will the people be wearing? What will the houses look like? What about the geography? Will there be trees and grass? You will be there shortly. Concentrate for a few moments. Let your imagination run freely...

Concentrate on your surroundings. See the colors of the rainbow so pretty in the sky. See it painted on the faces of people going by. See friends gathering, exchanging hugs, serene smiles, and peaceful looks. Study all of this and capture it by painting it on a huge canvass. When you are finished tell me what you see.

Jenny:

I see lots of trees, very green, meadows with real wooden fences. The sky is really blue with big white clouds. The people I see are smiling and all look very healthy. I see no trash, no cell phones, and no computers. The houses are made out of old looking brick and stone. It all has a European flavor. Some children are playing. The animals I see are dogs and sheep.

Wow! What does all this mean?

Steve T:

Well, I am not a dream interpreter Jenny and that is what you have experienced, a live dream. The important thing to know is that with your imagination, you can create what you want in life including thinking yourself thin. Would you like to create some more visualization scenarios in another session related to your future new look?

Jenny:

Absolutely. You are very good at this. This is great therapy!

Steve T:

It is easy to do with a willing and imaginative client, and that is you Jenny. There is a lady by the name of Shakti Gawain that has written a book called *Creative Visualization*. It is a very interesting and easy read. You may want to take a look at it.

Jenny:

I will.

REMAINDER OF SESSION SEVEN

With me asking leading questions, Jenny discussed the structures she has in place to help facilitate her weight loss. These include supportive people such as close friends and her church family, her employees, and even her dental patients. She has developed an exercise routine that is supported by friends and me, her coach, and others hold her accountable. Her food inventory at home and at the office has changed through absence of malice. In other words, there are no Reese's Peanut Buttercups or Lance crackers in sight. She views eating now in a different light. Her food attitude (fooditude) is changing.

SESSIONS EIGHT AND NINE

After nine weeks, Jenny has lost 24 pounds. Most of this is fat and she has been increasing muscle. Therefore, she looks like she has lost more than that. People, several people are beginning to notice. This is adding fuel to the fire for Jenny's desire to become the new her.

In these two sessions Jenny has solidified that she is a willing and dedicated client. Her attitude and desire to succeed are sterling.

Much of the discussion in these sessions have focused on exactly what Jenny is eating, how she is eating it (the eating process), when she is eating, and her portion sizes. There has been a lot of discussion about building a consistent eating lifestyle with the structure she has in place supporting her.

BETWEEN SESSION NINE AND TEN - A SUDDEN CHANGE!!!

A call to Steve in the evening, two days prior to their scheduled session

Jenny:

Steve, it's Jenny. I'm sorry to bother you but I had to call. Jenny breaks down. She is crying.

Steve T:

Jenny, what's wrong?

Jenny:

It's my Father. He passed away suddenly yesterday, and I didn't even get a chance to say goodbye. I feel like there was so much left to be said. Now I don't know what I can do.

Steve T:

Oh Jenny! I feel so bad for you. Yes, you definitely need someone to talk to. This would be a major set back for anybody. Losing a parent is one of the most difficult and emotional things anyone faces no matter when it happens.

Jenny, I am your coach and I have become your friend and I really want to help you. I appreciate your trust and confiding in me. You certainly did the right thing in calling me. I am hurting with you right now. Here is what I suggest to you. You need to talk with a grievance counselor. I think it would be best if you saw a counselor there in the Tampa area. However, if you wish, I will recommend someone you can counsel with by phone as we are doing. I will even pay for your session out of the proceeds you have given me if you are financially burdened.

Jenny:

Steve I am fine financially, but thanks. I have a lot of faith in what you say, so I will probably look for someone here. I am very emotional right now. I am afraid this is going to put a dent in my program.

Steve T:

A dent can be repaired Jenny. The program you have created for yourself will help you get through this. I am confident you will be able to stay in the steps. This newfound spirituality will aid you in dealing with all of life's situations, not just your eating.

Now for the moment this is a temporary setback. Why don't you seek counseling and we'll continue our sessions when you're ready. Would that work for you?

Jenny:

Yes, we will do that.

Steve T:

Okay, now that you have chosen to seek out an expert, I think it may help you to unload some of what you are feeling right now. I will be a willing listener if you wish to do so.

ONE YEAR LATER

Jenny, after fourteen months, lost 102 pounds, has dropped six dress sizes and is now wearing a size 12…well on her way to a 10. She only has twenty-eight more pounds to go to reach her goal weight of 135 pounds. She has just returned from her twenty-fifth high school reunion where she was the high school queen of her class. Everyone complimented her on how marvelous she looked and her husband was so proud of her. This made her feel good and full of confidence. She felt she could tackle just about anything. She is a leading advocate of health and wellness and is a frequent speaker in her community. She is feeling good about herself and about life.

Jenny did seek grief counseling to help her deal with her Father's death and she is feeling much better about the situation. She and her brother have become very close as they faced their loss together. She still sticks pretty close to The Three Bears Diet and is doing well. When she has minor setbacks, she calls Steve and they discuss how she can get back on track. Those calls are happening less frequently as time goes by.

CONCLUSION

The above illustration is a fictional account based upon real life coaching experiences. Although fictional, it is a very accurate depiction of what takes place during coaching sessions with stevetaylormyownweigh.com.

Emotional eating is a serious kind of addiction and should be treated as a disease. It takes will power, commitment and desire on the part of the person trying to lose the weight. But it also takes a support structure from understanding loved ones and trained experts who can help you discover the way to lose weight in a healthy way and fight through the set backs...and there will be setbacks. With the right mind-set and proper coaching, permanent weight loss is achievable.

Addendum 2
Glossary of Terms Used

Aerobic – A physical exercise is aerobic if it is designed to improve the cardiovascular system. This includes activities like running, swimming and walking.

Amino Acid – Acids that are building blocks for protein. Types of amino acid:
> - Essential amino acid – Protein building blocks, which the body cannot produce so they must be acquired from food.
> - Non-essential amino acid – A protein building block the body can synthesize.

Anaerobic – An anaerobic exercise does not promote the cardiovascular system. This includes activities like weight training or resistance training.

BMR (Basil Metabolic Rate) – The number of calories needed daily to maintain weight. It is determined based on gender, age, height, and weight as well as bone density, body frame and muscles.

Brain Flush – The Brain Flush is an exercise that helps identify the resentments and fear within our lives that may be the basis for emotional eating.

Carbohydrate – Carbohydrates are the main fuel source for the body. One gram of carbohydrate contains four calories. Glucose, the simplest carbohydrate is a must for brain cells, red blood cells, and is a main energy source for strenuous exercise. There are three kinds of carbs including sugars, starches, and fiber.

Emotional Eating – An eating disorder that causes a person to automatically and often unconsciously eat to deal with emotional pain.

Emotional Pain – A psychological or non-physical pain that is usually a derivation of or loss of one's self. Loss of one's self usually comes from the loss of another person, such as a death or a break-up in a relationship, or a conflict with another person.

Fat burner – A drug or supplement that can be purchased over the counter that claims to burn calories by increasing the rate of the body's metabolism.

Fats – Fats give texture and flavor to a lot of the foods we eat. There are nine calories per gram of fat. It is stored in fat cells, which help preserve body heat. It is also a source of energy. Types of fats:

-Monounsaturated Fat - Things like extra virgin olive oil, canola oil, peanut oil, avocados, almonds and walnuts.
-Polyunsaturated Fat – Examples include corn oil, sunflower oil, and safflower oil.
-Trans Fat – Fats that are considered unhealthy as they raise cholesterol and should be limited. Examples are cookies, donuts, shortening, cakes, crackers, and French fries.
-Unsaturated fats – Fats that become liquid at room temperature and are considered good because they lower bad cholesterol. May also help raise the good cholesterol (HDL).

Fiber - The part of the plant that cannot be digested by the body. It plays a crucial role in preventing the bacteria in our body from becoming toxic buildup. It is found in fruits, vegetables, and whole grains.

Fooditude – Food attitude or attitude about food.

Glycemic Index – A measurement of how each food impacts our blood sugar or blood glucose.

Morbidly Obese – A person who is 100 pounds or more overweight.

Obese – A person who is 20% or more overweight.

Portion Control – Eating only the amount of food needed by the body at the time.

Protein – Protein maintains muscle and some vital organs like the heart, kidneys, and lungs. There are four calories in each gram of protein. It creates antibodies that fight infection along with helping to form red blood cells.

The Six Food Groups – The six groups are dairy, fruits, vegetables, protein (meat and beans), oils or fats, and grains.